THE MASTERY OF CELTIC REIKI

BY

MARTYN PENTECOST

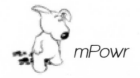 mPowr

First Published in Great Britain 2009 by mPowr (Publishing) Limited

www.mpowrpublishing.com
www.celtic-reiki.com

ISBN – 978-1-907282-02-7

Cover Design by Martyn Pentecost
mPowr Publishing 'Clumpy™' Logo by e-nimation.com
Clumpy™ and the Clumpy™ Logo are trademarks of mPowr Limited.

Made by Book Brownies!

Books published by mPowr Publishing are made by Book Brownies. A Book Brownie is about so high, with little green boots, a potato-like face and big brown eyes. These helpful little creatures tenderly create every book with kindness, care and a little bit of magic! Before shipping, a Book Brownie will jump into the pages—usually at the most gripping chapter or a part that pays particular attention to food—and stay with that book, always. This means that every mPowr Publishing book comes with added enchantment (and occasional chocolate smudges!) so that you get a warm, fuzzy feeling of love with the turn of every page!

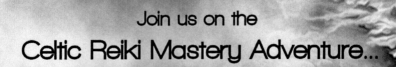

Join us on the
Celtic Reiki Mastery Adventure...

Free Mastery Training
when you purchase a
Celtic Reiki Mastery Book Bundle

www.celtic-reiki.com

For the Celtic Reiki Masters who have
cherished and respected our philosophies

Discover the Enchanted Realms of Celtic Reiki Mastery

Explore the magical path of Celtic Reiki Mystic and Realm Mastery at The Official Celtic Reiki Website. With information on various aspects of Celtic Reiki, a directory of Celtic Reiki Masters across the globe, and exclusive Realm Mastery Training with Martyn Pentecost, it is a wonderful online resource to begin your adventure.

If you're eager to begin your journey into the Sacred Grove, then join our community at www.celtic-reiki.com. A place where the Book Brownies live, the trees sing, and you'll always Be Enchanted!

www.celtic-reiki.com
The Official Celtic Reiki Website

Contents

INTRODUCTION

Humankind is currently experiencing a period of great change and evolution that is universally relevant. In this huge shift of paradigms, millions of people from different places and cultures are discovering an innovative approach to old wisdom; taking the beliefs of those who travelled this path before we came to be, and skimming away any of the obsolete philosophy and dogma that are so often attached to those beliefs.

We are waking up to the realisation that everybody is unique and has a very personal and individual authenticity. The historical tendency to convert or persuade other people to a particular edict or belief system is falling away and every one of us in this new paradigm is starting to express our own truth. The revelation in this wonderful new age is that we (for the most part) are not being burnt at the stake or crucified for doing so!

As if waking up to a bright new day, full of optimism for the future, each of us is now beginning to find an individual perspective on life and sharing this with others. By looking to the philosophies of yesterday and reimagining them in a more fluid, modern perspective, we are creating a remarkable synthesis. It is within this synthesis of science and spirituality, physical and ethereal, that we are finding truth and creating a 'Heaven on Earth' or what I personally call 'Viridia'.

For you, this may be another phase on a path you have been walking for a long time, or it could be the first tentative steps into a new realm of perception. I hope that whatever your path, this will be the start of an amazing new journey: the discovery of your own perfection and a sharing of that perfection with others.

I believe that somewhere within us, is the psychological equivalent of a big red button. At some point in a person's life, an event, situation or circumstance causes the button to be pushed and they wake up. Literally wake up to the illusion of the physical world. When this happens, there is no going back, no falling asleep, no matter how much we try. When my button was pushed, I awoke to a magical realm, guided by amazing individuals, such as Gill Edwards and her Living Magically books and James Redfield, author of the Celestine Prophecy series. Before long I was voraciously devouring knowledge about our new social and spiritual evolution.

I can remember doing palm and tarot readings in school for my fellow pupils. Dowsing with pendulums, astrology and seeing auras formed an integral part of my childhood. Yet, this new awakening was different; there was no need for the tools or gizmos that I had shunned in my scientific teens and early twenties. There was an organic simplicity and a very basic truth to the idea that there is more than just the solid world and rather than a distant perfection, ruled over by some unimaginable (but rather human in motivation) deity, this energetic realm was part of me. No, it was me and I was it.

This spiritual awakening to my own, special truth,

jolted me into a phantasmagorical adventure, where I came to experience moment after moment of spiritual revelation, filtered by the physical world. My reality shifted and I came to comprehend things in a very different way to other people. Very soon, I became aware that I was a pioneer and creator, although it took me the greater part of a decade to be comfortable with that definition.

One of my pioneering adventures was that of Celtic Reiki, an adaptation of what most people see as 'Reiki' practice into a different modality or 'flavour' of Reiki methodology. When I first began to teach Celtic Reiki, it was a simple practice with just under twenty essences and a wish that those who used those essences adapt and evolve the methods in accordance with their own truth.

As I expanded Celtic Reiki, growing it and reimagining it at regular intervals, I continued to encourage this integral sense of personal truth and the fluid framework. This, I believe is part of what makes Celtic Reiki so different and so valuable to those who work with it. It is your therapy, your art and yours to mould and evolve. I simply offer you a foundation, for you to construct the edifice of your choosing.

I have witnessed many people all over the world create buildings that are such beautiful works of art and value that I feel that I'm going to burst with joy. I have also seen people pull up the foundations and offer piles of bricks.

It was these isolated instances of Celtic Reiki (mal) practice that spurred me to act. I totally and absolutely believe in a flexibility of practice in Celtic Reiki that enables people to speak and act on their own core truths. I also recognise the right of those wanting to learn and be treated with Celtic Reiki to get what they expect and have some ability to verify what they are taught against a series of standards and guidelines.

An analogy of how I see this in connection to Celtic Reiki teaching and practice is that of a person coming to a store to buy some food. In my store I would want to provide them with seeds, gardening equipment, fishing rods and livestock so that they could grow and rear their own food in the future. I would also throw in enough food to sustain the person until they could be self-sufficient.

The majority of Celtic Reiki Masters uphold that ethos and provide ways of empowering their students. Some only provide the tools, some the seeds, some only provide the food itself. All of these are still what the person, coming to the store, wants. It is the stores that provide balloons and pieces of carpet that concern me. These items have their usages, but they are not what the customer ordered! Celtic Reiki Masters, in my opinion, have personal truth as their innate birthright; they also need to ensure that their clients get what they ask for and that anything that is not, at a foundation level 'Celtic Reiki' should not be presented as such.

Hence, I decided to write three books on the Celtic Reiki system and that each of these would reflect a specific element of the practice. One would be a funny and poignant history of the creation of Celtic Reiki, told through the stories I collected along the way; the anecdote and the allegory.

Next would be a luxurious guide book, a keepsake of all the major philosophies and essences of Celtic Reiki. And, finally, this book, which I see as a progression of the other two, aimed at anybody who is a Celtic Reiki Master, Practitioner, Trainee, or simply has an interest in what it's all about!

This book of Mastery would not only build on the principles of the other two books and the actual courses and seminars; it would be a call to action for everybody connected to Celtic Reiki, a way of us all gathering around a huge campfire and sharing a tale or two together as a family. Those tales would enable us to step back into the world, now with a renewed sense of vigour, direction and purpose.

If you are a Celtic Reiki Master, Practitioner, or Student, it's my heartfelt wish that this book offer inspiration and sparks of insight to help you grow your practice and seminars. If you are exploring the idea of learning Celtic Reiki yourself or would like Celtic Reiki treatments, this book will show you what to expect and how to assess the right Master for your own needs.

I have always seen Celtic Reiki as a gift, given by the trees, which over time, I have defined and sculpted according to my own sense of innate truth. The results of which, I wanted to share with others, so that they might discover their own truth and wisdom. I perceive this book as a gift also. It is my way of saying thank you to everybody who has created joy through their Celtic Reiki practice and teachings. It is my way of showing gratitude to you, my fellow Master, traveller, explorer and friend.

May the journey that we share in these pages lead us on to a tangible and lasting sense of bliss at all the exciting voyages we have yet to uncover.

The Foundations of Celtic Reiki

Celtic Reiki is a popular modality of Energy Therapy that was created from a synthesis of two traditional philosophies. The first of these philosophies is derived from the Shinto belief of everything being created from a force known as Ki. One of the facets of this Ki is Reiki, which has the ability to heal and balance the other types of Ki.

The second philosophy is a modern perspective, evolved from that of the Celtic people of Western Europe, which holds the natural world in very high esteem. The Celts believed that the trees were sacred and based much of their way of life in relation to our tree friends. By combining the two viewpoints, we can synthesise the innate forces of the Universe with the vibrations of trees. When doing this, you can work therapeutically and with manifestation techniques to help others and yourself.

Over time, the philosophies of Celtic Reiki have made many an evolutionary step. At times, in the methods of practice, and at others with the depth of knowledge that is not necessarily sourced from a Celtic perspective, but is actually derived from the wisdom of the trees: the wisdom that originally inspired the Celts and created many paths of faith and belief.

Since I started to teach Celtic Reiki, so much has happened in the world and we have all evolved beyond the original scope of the practice. For my own part, I have changed in virtually every way since my first experience with the first Celtic Reiki vibration. These changes have not only offered me insights into the practical and material aspects of Celtic Reiki that needed to change but have also created such an integral link between the trees and myself that I have been given so much more than I ever thought possible: wisdom that I now share with you.

Celtic Reiki is the result of my own journey through energy work and, partially for this reason, I have previously chosen to write about Celtic Reiki in the style of a personal story or journal rather than a work of reference. In my book, Stories from the Sacred Grove, I relate the incident with the Ash who advised me not to create dogma in the practice of Celtic Reiki.

It was this beautiful Ash tree (who, incidentally had a very good sense of humour), who explained, the thing I wanted most for Celtic Reiki could never be attained whilst I continued to make the biggest mistake of all. The one thing I have always loved about energetic therapy is that it is such a personal and individual practice that can be adapted to the needs of the individual and their existing beliefs.

As each and every person learns, practises and eventually teaches Celtic Reiki to others, it evolves and becomes fluid – it changes. From the very outset, I asked that those who used it should develop Celtic Reiki further. As I originally offered an 'incomplete' system, this soon happened as Celtic Reiki Masters across the globe filled in the gaps and brought the 'missing' vibrations home.

Yet Celtic Reiki did not evolve for many years – It found stasis and changed only within that stasis: ever different, but never moving in synch with the Universe and the massive changes that are occurring in our world. Why? The responsibility is mine and mine alone – I taught Celtic Reiki in a definitive and prescriptive manner.

Having studied various forms of Reiki practice for many years, I was guided to act with the natural world. When working with Reiki to help Animals, Plants, Trees, Rivers, Lakes, the Oceans and the Earth itself, I found that everything has a distinct vibration – each variety of rock, each stream, each type of flower has its own unique perspective of energy. I would sometimes lose myself so deeply in the sensations, derived from this energy that I could recreate the vibrations during Reiki self-treatments.

Late one winter's day, whilst on a visit to Wales, I discovered a huge Silver Fir tree that had been split in two by a recent lightning strike. One half was still firmly rooted upright, while the other half was lying on the ground, dying. As I walked up to the tree, I could sense the immense loss felt by the upright section and an urgency of the fallen half that was completely separated from the standing section.

I connected to Reiki and started to treat the standing section but could feel a resistance, so I asked what I should do. After several attempts, I finally began to work by placing one hand on the fallen half and one on the standing half. As I did this, it felt as if I became part of the tree, completely absorbed and assimilated by its vibration, its 'essence'.

This experience was unlike anything I had felt before – the essence of the tree – its knowledge, its force, its wisdom and its love. When it felt as if the process had reached a natural conclusion, I started to work with the standing section of tree. It was an amazing experience, being enveloped by the gratitude and love of the healthy section of this massive tree.

As the energy faded, I was able to return to the usual Usui Reiki and work on healing the tree's broken trunk. I was overwhelmed by an inner voice, which said the tree was very grateful for my assistance and would allow me to use its vibration to help others. I was instructed that I could help people to 'see' with that particular type of energy vibration.

As I left the site, I touched the fallen part of the tree and felt very little, as if the consciousness, the life of the tree had gone, leaving only the wood.

This led me on a further journey of discovery – for the Celts believed the Silver Fir represented the ability to see over long distances – to view the horizon – to 'see'. I began to understand the meaning of the tree in Wales and the wisdom of the Celtic people. I now firmly believe that they knew the essence of each tree and plant type – so complete was their relationship with the Earth that they were sensitive to the resonance and the energy around them, harnessing and using this energy to assist them in life.

I decided to work with other types of tree to see if there was continuity in this pattern, so I set out on my quest, starting with the Yew Tree. I had a chance to visit a cemetery in Gloucestershire, where 99 Yew trees grew – several attempts have been made to plant a one-hundredth tree, but the tree always dies. Here I found resonance with a particular Yew tree that permitted me to work with his essence, during which time he informed me that he would "guide me beyond endings". I started to work with the essence 'Ioho' – finding that it helped me to cope with any type of change or loss: Speeding up the recovery process or guiding me through rough patches with greater ease.

I continued to develop Celtic Reiki with the help of many trees and plants in this way, guided by the wisdom of the Celts to choose locations and types of essence. Having studied many books on the subject, I started to use the Celtic alphabet or 'Ogham' in order to 'trigger' essences and create an easier way for people to use many different vibrations if they choose to. This process of triggering is used in many esoteric practices as a way of intending the connection to a particular facet of energy or perspective. Akin to the emotional attachments we form with certain words or names, the use of a symbol in energy work is believed to offer a way of defining energy in usable 'chunks'.

Much of Celtic Reiki was based on the themes that ran through historical information about the Celts as well as comparisons between each source and the individual tree essences. It seemed that the information written about the Celts tied in with the findings from testing the essences in practice!

As time went on however, I slowly came to realise that by working with Celtic Reiki through the eyes of traditional writing and modern references was actually limiting the beliefs of the system. In fact, basing Celtic Reiki practice on any historical method would limit it. So I went back to the drawing board and started to rework my original system to something that was very different, primarily due to the way in which the course was written.

In later styles of Celtic Reiki, I attempted to create a journal feel to the findings for each Ogham Trigger and the essence attached to it. I worked purely on my findings from treating people, client feedback and intuition, trying not to refer to any texts or writing. What I found was a system that was truer and that appeared to be more like the Celtic healing practices. It was also these revised practices that led me on to many more discoveries and magical enhancements, hence enabling a very different and powerful form of energetic art.

Looking back, I realised how my desire to keep revising the methodology stemmed from a need to maintain its fluidity and to keep the system alive through change, as opposed to letting it become dogmatised or stagnant. The Celts never wrote their wisdom down and it is only in pictures and conjecture that we can guess at the form of their spiritual beliefs. Having looked for a foundation in writing, I had been using the essences from a narrow perspective – by writing a journalised system I was offering my perspective of Celtic Reiki.

Following this methodology, I understood that in many ways Celtic Reiki should not be written down – it should be conducted as a verbal practice, passed down orally from teacher to student, although as this is not feasible in our modern world, I maintained the journal feel to my notes, articles and books; usually offering suggestions on how to the use of the vibrations and recommending techniques. I developed unusual forms of information transmission, such as energy encoding and calibration techniques. These did not involve written forms of communication, but vibrational, energy communication we shall investigate later in this book.

My voyage has become one that has led me to ancient woods and wide moors, where the trees often have a deep mistrust of humankind for the ravages we have inflicted on the natural world. As a gaining of trust and a mutual bonding has forged relationships with these creatures, I have established a deeper connection to them than ever before. I now view these fellow travellers as friends, some loving and caring, some austere and courageous, others are protective and nurturing. All are wise and carry with them a knowledge that connects us to the wisdom of our past, the choices of our present and the foresight of our futures.

The assorted trees that have lived on this earth longer than any of us, are capable in their own unique ways of an undying love, an unbreakable strength, and an unquestionable knowledge. They are also capable of harsh judgment, deep suspicion and a horrible pain, so foreboding that we cannot imagine it. It is this that makes the Celtic Reiki essences we use so powerful. For the trees and plants applied in the Celtic systems know our most thoroughly hidden and darkest places, the extremes of our fears, our innermost secrets and most truly embarrassing moments, because they too have experienced them and gone beyond them to a place of understanding and empowerment. By working with their essences we can turn our dark to light and find the love, strength and wisdom of the world.

The techniques I developed to harvest the vibrations of plants and trees have been adapted for use in many therapies though they remain very much part of Celtic Reiki, which continues to evolve and become of greater importance in the responsibilities of humankind than I ever imagined.

As such, many have adapted and re-purposed Celtic

Reiki into other forms of therapy and many different forms of 'Celtic' energy are available on the Internet and elsewhere. This is at the heart of my discoveries as, for something to evolve, it must become many different things. I do believe that for a practice, philosophy or method to be true to itself and maintain its integrity, there does need to be a very particular definition and it is for this reason I have offered a framework in this book. What follows are not 'hard and fast' rules that need to be 'obeyed'; they are recommendations and a snapshot of what Celtic Reiki encompasses as a therapy.

The various essences mentioned in this book are from my own collection of essences; they are gifts from friends that I have made along the way. Passed on through processes known as 'Orientation' and 'Calibration', students of Celtic Reiki experience an amazing, spiritual awakening as they alter their awareness and learn how to use the essences at a physical level of awareness. Each essence offers a very worthwhile and valuable set of energy frequencies that can help create a huge spectrum of intents and purposes. However, to really experience and totally understand the nature of the Celtic wisdom and the vibrations of the plants around us, it is down to the individual practitioners to build their own knowledge; working with trees and other beings, to assist and repay what we have been given.

By working with the essences at their source, the Celtic Reiki Master can realise something far greater than I can ever offer: an understanding that they have endeavoured for personally, learned by their own means and contribution to nature. Celtic Reiki is the title by which people recognise the art, but the energy each Master works with, the lessons they teach, the passion they feel are created by each individual and, just like the trees that helped to make this therapy, that is the most important thing each Master can give to the world – uniqueness!

The Principles of Trees

Have you ever wondered why the tree that grows in the shade, destined to live a life of darkness, never relinquishes her quest to reach towards the light? Did you notice how the tree that has been cut back to a mere stump will often shoot tiny new branches in an attempt to live just a little while longer? Do you ever stop for a moment and question the inner motivations of a tree that has fallen in a storm as he continues his growth, as long as a single root is left in the Earth?

A tree whose leaves are burnt by the howling wind will simply grow his branches in the direction, away from the fiercest of gales. The tree that is baked by the most dehydrating rays of Grandmother Sun will send his roots deeper into the ground in search of moisture. The tallest tree in the forest does not stop growing because she is higher than her brothers and sisters.

Now imagine what it would be like if trees adopted the behaviours of so many humans in the Western world. If a tree refused to produce leaves because, as an acorn, his mother dropped him in a patch of dense thicket, or if a tree refused to drink water because it was too cold or the soil was a tad on the sandy side. What would happen if a tree refused to grow taller, because its branches might hinder those, less fortunate from growing? And can you comprehend a tree deciding to die and rot away because it was told to, by another?

No, trees do not stop growing if the conditions are not perfectly suited to their needs. They don't feel embarrassment because their branches have become gnarled or their trunks have been scarred. Trees cherish every moment of life on Father Earth. They learn their ancestry and strive towards the light every day.

I am aware that I may be over-simplifying things by comparing the life of a tree to that of a human, with all our complexity and intelligence, however just take a moment to ponder this: what would our lives be like if rather than trying to be the best, have the most, procrastinate the longest, or expecting others to do things on our behalf, we spent every day wringing every last of drop of joy from our lives as possible? What if we basked on sunny days, drunk thirstily when it rained, if the wind burnt us we found another direction to grow in and if the unthinkable happened, we simply started anew with what we had left?

I've never met a tree that blamed her neighbours for growing too close, or a sapling that blamed his elders for blocking out the sunlight. Trees have no time for blame or giving away their power. Every tree is focussed on one thing and one thing alone – the experience of life.

There is no doubt that we are staggering in how much more progressive we are than our tree friends. We have achieved wondrous things within the context of our human perspective. Rockets to the moon, medicine and the Internet do not hold much fascination for trees, whose attention is usually on growth, experience and a sense of being a vital part of the journey through time.

If a person attempted to live as simply as the tree,

our complex world would simply move beyond them, because our growth as a species is outwards, rather than up and down – we are expansive creatures and therefore our needs are different. I believe that we do require more from life than the small satisfactions of a tree. Yet, a variety of aspects remain the same – like trees, we grow, physically, experientially, spiritually. We may start out on the journey of our lives in glorious sunlight, sometimes shrouded in darkness. Disaster can strike at times, situations and circumstances may hinder us, and we all exist in the same physical world. Both trees and humans are custodians of this world; we have the task of keeping him and all that live upon him, safe, nurtured and supported as best we can.

These common bonds mean that we have a lot to learn from how our tree companions approach each new day with all its challenges and treasures

An Ancient Language

It was a hot summer's day several years ago when I was sitting on a train, pondering the ability to mimic exactly the vibrations of a tree. I was in the very early stages of creating Celtic Reiki and it fascinated me, how we could capture a vibration and use it without the need for a physical 'hook' to attach it to.

Homeopaths use remedies in the form of tablets, soaked in a potentised solution, which retains the vibration of a specific object, or substance. It is possible, however, for a homeopath to prescribe these vibrations without the use of remedies, purely because they have had contact with the remedy and 'remember' its vibration. As a teacher of Energy Entrainment, this sparked my curiosity and I was internalising how a person could 'take' the vibration of a tree for this purpose.

A flash of inspiration fell into my head at that moment, it was one of many encouraging thoughts that filled my head around this time. I did not understand many of those thoughts fully, but knew at an integral level that it would all make sense eventually.

At this time, I was working very intuitively, following what some might call my higher guidance. It seemed like such a long way from my training in Cosmology and Quantum Physics and yet, I was soon to realise that both the disciplines of science and spirituality would create a synthesis that would revolutionise my way of working in therapy and life.

Through the training in scientific theory, combined with energy work, I was able to interpret the higher wisdom I experienced into practical, physical systems. I was so passionate about this adventure playground of energy work that I created several forms of Reiki modality, these included Karmic Reiki, which has now evolved into Karmic Regression Therapy and Crystal Reiki, (now used as part of the Celtic Reiki ethos). With several, very different and (at the time) unusual ways of working with Reiki as a form of treatment, I decided to move on to other forms of therapy, such as the Viridian Method.

Yet Celtic Reiki kept calling to me and over the years I spent a great deal of time growing, nurturing and expanding the system. It was during these precious moments that I discovered the underlying nature of the system, not only as Celtic Reiki, but in the form of Celtic spirituality and as Reiki methodology, as well.

The connection, created between tree and human, or human and energy is not a give-and-take scenario. There is no transferral of energy or offering of oneself. The connections we create are communications in a strange and unfamiliar tongue. For instance, imagine asking a person for directions to a place in the local area. They would respond by explaining the steps in getting from here to there; starting at 'a' and ending at 'b'.

If we understand that the vibrational perspective of a tree can help heal a disease or trauma, then what we perceive is the method of using the vibrational pattern of a tree to take us from dis-ease to ease, pain to joy, not-having to having. These directions of how to achieve the 'state of being' we desire does not take the form of words or a linguistic language, it is a language of potential or energy.

In the same way that waves of sound carry a voice from one person's mouth to another's ears, or in which analogue radio waves once transmitted television pictures from broadcaster to TV sets across many nations, by working with the vibration of a tree (or other form of vibrational energy) we are reproducing lost and ancient languages in our own bodies and minds.

The ancient Kotodama are a set of monosyllabic sounds that enable those who evoke them to 'become the energy' particular to that sound. For example, the Kotodama 'su' was said to be the sound that created the Universe. Music has often been used to change mood or create a state of awareness. Both sound and light are used as forms of therapy and how many people would say they feel better when the sun is shining?

Light, sound, vibrations are communication in (mostly) non-verbal forms. Reiki, for me, is also a form of communication – of compassion, love, joy, bliss, and well-being, (amongst other things). The different styles of Reiki practice, I view as dialects that appeal to different people. So some prefer the traditional Eastern views of Usui Reiki, some the Huna principles of Karuna Reiki, some the modern ethos of vReiki and many, the deep resonance of the Celts in Celtic Reiki.

Over the years, I have taught Celtic Reiki to those with Druidic and Wiccan training, many who feel passionately about the natural world, people from all over the globe, looking for connection to their Celtic ancestry, Usui Reiki Masters, Therapists, and people who just love trees.

For each person that I speak to, there is a common theme of Celtic Reiki 'speaking' to people with a resonance and connection that they have never experienced before. I believe this language is of the trees and beyond that: the Earth.

Our Mother, our Father Earth is calling to us in our own unique tongue. Reconnecting to those who are willing to listen and offering us a deeply personal experience of coming home. The language is slightly different for every person, yet it is always just what we need to hear or discover.

As Celtic Reiki has developed, adapted and evolved over the years, it has grown from a 'give-and-take approach', where tree and human exchange vibrations and transformed into an expression of one's truth. In the origination and adaptation processes, I have focussed less and less on the prescriptive, highly defined approach of the early days and have attempted to create an art-form that is about expression and the communication of love and companionship between the natural world, trees and humans alike.

From Celtic Reiki as a therapy to a lost art to a language (of vibration), the methodology has become finely nuanced and yet, absolutely vast in its encompassment. From a handful of treatment methods, basic attunements and under twenty Tree Essences, the system consists of Realms, Avatars, Lores, Archetypes, Ranges of Essences and many, many stories!

This is hardly surprising, as from the very beginning we used the Ogham or Celtic alphabet as a way of accessing the essences and communicating Celtic Reiki from one person to another. Even in the early days, we could spell out treatments, using the letters of the Ogham to form 'energy words'.

As I use the English language to convey the methods and practices of the Celtic Reiki Master to you now, I hope that you may hear the lost language softly in the background; calling to you a remembrance of who you are and your innate power as part of the Earth, the Universe.

As you read on, it is my intention not simply to list the methods of Mastery (although I shall be doing this also), I want to show you a glimpse of what it is to be a Celtic Reiki Master. Not simply a Practitioner, Mentor and Teacher, but of one who walks the Earth, deeply connected and whispering in an ancient tongue – a Lost Language that is waiting to be heard again.

WHAT'S IN A NAME?

The title 'Celtic Reiki' and its descriptive influences on how people perceive the practice is much debated. While some understand the term to be a symbiosis of 'Celitc' Philosophy and 'Reiki' Practice, others suggest that the term denotes the 'Reiki' of the 'Celtic' People. Some ask, "Did the Celts use Reiki?" and then there are those who state "But Usui never visited Britain!" There are people who have hypothesised that Celtic Reiki is actually a rediscovery of Nearth, the Celt-equivalent of Ki, and others take the approach that "it's just Reiki with a twist".

My belief is that all of these statements are true and yet, they are all not true too! The challenge of any hybrid philosophy is carving a niche for itself in a world where people have a tendency to feel comfortable with familiarity. I also found comfort in the simple analogy of a tree's perspective of Reiki for many years – I could recognise the idea of a tree reflecting Reiki to me, because it was congruent with my schema of Usui Reiki practices. Over the years of working with Celtic Reiki, my beliefs have adapted and changed considerably, not only of how I perceived Celtic Reiki, but due to how Celtic Reiki perceived me.

Both the traditions of the Celts and Shinto principles of Ki have, at their very foundations, a truth that is beyond space and time. This truth is infinite and eternal and it is these very definitions that create such difficulties for us.

The Celts' respect for the Earth (as 'part of it' as opposed to 'masters of it') is so relevant to many people today because, in our ecologically damaged and disrespected world, we yearn to reclaim our love of the Earth. We are the Earth and at some deep-rooted place, inside each of us, every tree and animal killed is a part of us dead, the damage to the atmosphere is dis-ease within, the terror and fear we feel for each other is the Earth rousing and preparing for a great, levelling change. We know we need to act differently, to break free from our habitual hatred and discover compassion once again.

Thus, we look back to the last time humans (en masse) were so in sync with their nature and imbue those people with the qualities we so desire now. The issue is that the Celts were not the peace-loving custodians we romanticise them into today. Without the modern, cultural principles and technology we rely on and to a certain extent, take for granted, they had to survive in the face of dangers we cannot comprehend and problems we have never known.

With these challenges the defining factor in a cultural behaviour, the Celtic tribes were often brutal in ways that are quite chilling by modern standards. Therefore in modern society, we may feel the need to love and respect the Earth as demonstrated by our Celtic ancestors, however the need to disembowel each other over the roots of trees to appease the forest deities may not be such a welcome reintroduction into elementary schools!

When we feel nostalgic for the Celtic perspective, it is not a need to be Celtic or even to emulate them – it is the pang of recognition that to survive in harmony with our own essential being, we need to reconnect to the truth that exists at the core of our Celtic lineage.

When we turn to the principles of Ki, we discover a truth that encompasses the nature of all things, not only that of the Earth. This ancient ideology can be traced back even further than that of the Celts and symbolises a balancing dynamic that creates harmony and equilibrium.

If the Celtic philosophies were centred on the Earth, contractive into the physical world, of birth and Beith and what some may term as 'feminine', the essence of Ki wisdom is 'Spirit'-centred, expansion into the Universe/Source, of death and Ioho, the 'masculine'. Both the Celtic ethos and that of Ki are cyclic, with each turning back upon themselves – with birth comes the inevitable death and through death we attain rebirth.

In my book 'Stories from the Sacred Grove', I explore the very nature of Ki, the facets and dynamics they create, from Shinki (the Divine) to Kekki (the Blood). In a Western context these ideals are mostly ignored in Reiki practices, because they are, initially, very different from our own cultural context. With time and deeper insight, their logic and truth can be seen in so many threads of Western spirituality and ideology. The idea of energy manifest as the solid world, the experience of isolation and reconnection, how we interact to create a plethora of emotions, art, philosophy and religion, and so on. Yet, within the context of the Ki perspective, there is much that does not fit with the modern perspective and requires adaptation to a contemporary mindset.

Thus, when we speak of Reiki in the context of Celtic Reiki, I believe this balancing and healing force is contextual to the modern world, as opposed to being 'the Reiki' spoken of in Shinto, or indeed, by Mikao Usui. Now some may find this disheartening, however Reiki in the perspective of 19th Century person would not be as effective for us as that defined for the 21st Century situations we encounter on a daily basis. Of course, it is important to mention here that the 'truth' of Ki is beyond context, however, in the physical world where we form a connection between body and Ki, it requires definition and it is this definition that creates the effectiveness of Reiki practices in any given circumstance.

Imagine that you are having a conversation with a person who believes the world is flat. You may know what exists beyond the horizon, although this may differ from the other person's concept of the world. Your version of the world and theirs are different and while each viewpoint works adequately for each of you, individually, would you trust a map they offer you as accurate? Well, if you a navigating around Europe, this map would probably serve your needs very well. If you wanted to circum-navigate the globe, perhaps not.

Now imagine what your map would do for them! It would either be completely unacceptable or it would blow their mind to such an extent that they transcend their current worldview. In the case of the latter, they would have to construct a very different set of parameters of what they thought they knew. This could be seen as an analogy of Reiki – there is a truth, though we only ever know refinements (or varieties) of that truth.

Thus, Celtic Reiki is neither Celtic nor Reiki in the simple, contextual meaning and it is both. I view the methods of Celtic Reiki as a mode of transportation to other philosophies, perspectives, abilities, and states of being; Celtic, Japanese, and Universal. I could suggest, therefore, that the Celtic and the Reiki explains more about the people who use it than the focus of that usage!

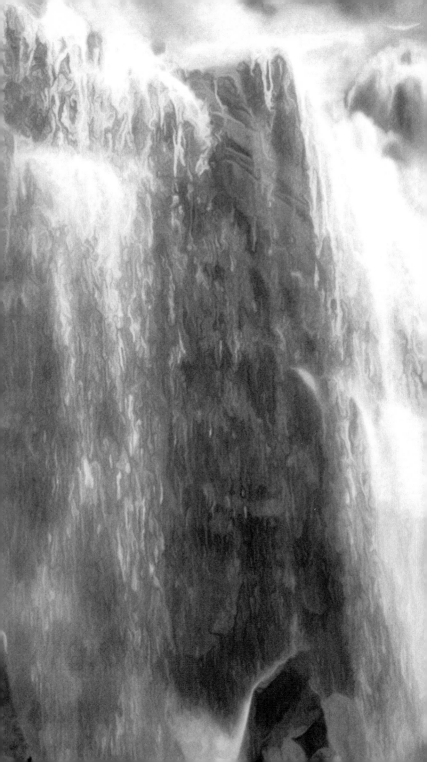

THE FIVE REALMS OF CELTIC REIKI

In the later adaptations of Celtic Reiki methodology we mould our practices within one of five dynamics or Realms, which refines treatments and alters the end results. This could be looked upon in the same way that sound is affected by different environments – a tune in the shower sounds different to that sung outside. Reiki is also changed, not by environment, but through the dynamic it is associated with.

The five Realms are:

- The Woodland Realm
- The Standing Stones
- The Celestial Realm
- The Mountain Range
- The Furthest Ocean

In many ways, the Realms represent the most startling change in Celtic Reiki Mastery, because they move us beyond the Woodland and provide a carriage, upon which we can travel to new layers of practice, based firmly in the natural world at a Universal level. The reasoning behind the creation of the Realms, was to instil an autonomy within the philosophy of Celtic Reiki; preserving the Celtic wisdom and grounding in tree essences, whilst also giving us the scope of additional essences and procedures that create a blossoming in the range of our techniques, tools, and methods.

Thus, Celtic Reiki is no longer a therapy, self-development tool, or Reiki practice – the days of simply listing essences to form a treatment are resigned to the earliest forms of practice. Now, Celtic Reiki is an art form, of sculpting essences, honing their effect and aesthetic, shaping the energy of everything we do, and embracing a range of philosophies that encompass ancient wisdom that dates back 5,000 years.

The best way I can describe how the Realms achieve such a huge surge of expansion is to imagine our practice in and through time as a time-line with a circle placed upon it. Now imagine that this circle is located at a point when Mikao Usui created the Usui Reiki Ryoho. As Hayashi and Takata adapted the practice the circle expands into the each passing moment: the leading edge of the circle always current and existing in the modern time. The circle, therefore grows with time and expands to the sides; I view this as range of treatment, which is why Usui Reiki practice often incorporates unrelated practices – to fill the gaps created by the expansion. To keep the ever-increasing circle full of wisdom, there has to be some form of adaptation to make it 'fit' with a modern perspective. Without this adaptation, we actually need to travel backwards in perspective to meet the requirements of the circle – this is why those who refuse to adapt a practice (the purists) lose connection between the way a practice achieves results and the reality of the world around them.

Imagine a methodology that was created in the 19th Century, for the dis-eases of the time. Without any adaptation, that method would be wonderful when working with people who have typhoid or small-pox, but not as equipped to deal with HIV/AIDS or Crystal Meth addiction! When the ethos of ancient tradition is not adapted for modern needs it is the practitioner who shifts their perspective, as opposed to the practice that caters to the perspective of the practitioner. This does not mean that traditions have to be altered beyond recognition to become relevant in modernity – they simply need some shifting of purpose, incorporation of widely accepted, current perspectives and some gentle removal of any dogma that has found its way into the tradition.

Now visualise what occurred at the point of Celtic Reiki creation – the circle was not only pushed backwards through our timeline to the Celtic period of European history, it was pushed forward to encompass a modern perspective of the practice needs, philosophy and outcomes. The circle expanded at the modern-edge and at the opposing, historical-edge. This not only enabled the integration of greater wisdom (both traditional and modern), it also offered us a greater range of practice – represented by the two side edges of the circle. Hence, the therapy, became manifestation tool, psychic-ability enhancer, lost language and connector to our Earth.

Our visualisation does not end here, though. Now imagine that rather than a circle on a line, it is a sphere that traverses time. Like a giant, inflatable ball, with a string through the centre, representing our perception of time. Now, the adaption of old traditions to a modern perspective, not only expands the relevance of a method in the past, present and future, as well as the range of practice and theory – it also increases the depth and integrity of the wisdom (the bottom of the sphere) and the spiritual growth (the top of the sphere). Any and every adaptation into the past and future creates overall growth in every direction.

A simple, rigid circle offers a set level of results, fixed in time and attitude. A constantly adapted and expanding sphere creates exponential, overall evolution...not only of a method, but also of the Master of the method. The adaptation of Celtic Reiki practices to encompass the Shinto and Tao philosophies, pushed our sphere to an even more expansive range of practice, higher spiritual growth, and greater depth of integrity. This expansion enabled the addition of Non-Celtic Tree Essences, Woodland Essences, and Elemental Essences; the latest expansion enabled the inclusion of even more wisdom and ability.

The pushing back of philosophy into the past created the need for the Celtic Reiki Realms; frameworks or definitions that enable the Master to sort or classify her practice into manageable areas of knowledge and experience. There is currently a greater depth of wisdom, a larger range of treatment styles, a wider degree of uses, a higher level of results and a more-encompassing integrity to Celtic Reiki study, practice and mastery than the majority of Usui Reiki styles available.

Each of the five Realms is immersive and vast in the effects it creates, for you are no longer conducting treatments or practices in your everyday environment – by using the Realms, you are shifting your awareness to places of awe-inspiring complexity and reality. Celtic Reiki Masters are taught how to enter the Realms and work from within their dynamics, however we shall briefly examine each of the five Realms here, as an introduction to their contrasting natures

The Woodland Realm

The Woodland Realm represents the Spatial Element (Space) and envelopes the Celtic Reiki Tree Essences, both Celtic and Non-Celtic varieties. The experienced practitioner or master will align with the Woodland Realm before any practice that involves tree essences, although a natural alignment will occur through the use of the appropriate essence or essences.

When using tree essences for treatment, manifestation or some other purpose, the dynamic tends towards a expansion, where both the originator of the essence and the focus expand and develop. So, the master/practitioner and client/subject of the practice both evolve and grow by using the essences.

The tree essences of Celtic Reiki are akin to the woodland or forest, each essence representing a tree or shrub that interacts with its neighbours and seeks to grow and develop, both individually and as part of a group.

By attuning their perspective to the Woodland Realm, the originator defines the desired outcome as that of the woodland. This realm represents a sacred, peaceful and enchanted place where the subject can heal, learn, explore, discover, create, relax, and find spiritual awakening.

My personal view of the Woodland Realm is that of a sanctuary of the body; a place for the weary traveller to rest a while, to take nourishment and time to heal themselves, nurture their strength, and invigorate their energy, in preparation for the onward journey. The holistic layers of the self (our emotional, psychological and spiritual layers) are also empowered through the physical (spatial) world.

It is often said that Celtic Reiki uses Reiki "channelled through the Earth" or from the Earth, particularly when referring to the tree essences. This is slightly misleading from my perspective, because I believe that the Celtic Reiki Tree Essences work with all four elements, through our spatial perspective.

A tree grows in the Earth, drinks water, processes

the air, and feeds on sunlight (fire) – it does so in space and time, hence the foundation ethos of the Woodland Realm as a spatial dynamic through which we create a range of powerful results with our tree friends.

The Standing Stones

The Standing Stones are of the Earth, yet they create a connection to the Celestial Realm and to the air. In so many ways the stones are akin to the trees, so it is fitting that this Realm encompasses the crystal and mineral essences, as well as drawing from Nordic theology; a counterpart to that of the Celts. The Runic symbolism that is associated with these essences mirrors the Ogham and, offers a symmetrical beauty to the tree and crystal essence use.

Although there are many connections and similarities between the tree and the stone, their consciousnesses are different; the stone awareness exists upon distant, intangible layers of perception, way beyond the usual perception of people. Crystals display the three requirements to be classed as 'living'; they grow, the reproduce and they communicate – even at a distance. If a crystal is struck, other crystals in the vicinity will display a change in vibration also.

These qualities offer the attuned Celtic Reiki Master a vast insight into the Earth at a deep level of perception. The wisdom of the trees represents lifetimes of hundreds of years, thousands in terms of the Lost Language.

Yet, the stones represent millions of years of life, which extends to billions in some essences and through the foundation layers of every Nordic Stone Essence. Therefore, if the trees represent the ever-changing, fleeting moment of experience; stone essences provide a deep-rooted grounding that transcends time. There are still adaptations, but these are so distended over time, as to be indiscernible without drastic alterations in perception.

A remarkable aspect of the Standing Stones is they form gateways between worlds. When a crystal communicates with another it does so instantaneously and over huge distances. This 'phenomenon' has caused much deliberation in the scientific community, launching many an inquisitive mind to theorise of different dimensions to achieve these most amazing results. What is important in a Celtic Reiki perspective is the concept that if crystals communicate instantly across thousands of miles, they can most certainly do it over interstellar distances!

The Celestial Realm

The Celestial Realm has many connections with the element of Air, both in the physical sense of 'up in the air' and the ethereal sense of air as spiritual belief and what lies beyond the Earth. The Stellar Essences (planets, stars and constellations) are equated with the Celestial, which also represents the connection to otherworldly places, far off locations and the 'Stargate Essence'.

The dynamic of the Celestial Realm is transcendence, for it exists beyond the movements of three-dimensional perception. There are no paths or linear journeys in the action of this Realm. Here we transcend our physical Earth and come to understand the layers of perception, which exist beyond our human comprehension. The Celestial Realm is truly alien in its very fabric, not only because it is not of the Earth, but it is not of regular human perception.

We can best understand the Celestial Realm and the essences it encompasses, by comparison to the Woodland Realm and our tree essences. For trees and humans alike, the Earth is our home and all that we have ever known in physical terms. With so many common points of reference, when we harvest or connect to tree essences the perspectives mingle and it can be challenging to decipher which perspective we are working from. There are so many truly incomprehensible aspects to the Celestial Realm that it becomes very apparent when a perspective is human or alien. We each have our own perspective of the constellation Orion, for example, though as soon as you experience the Orion Essence from a non-terrestrial perspective, it will transcend anything you have ever known.

It is an interesting element of this Realm that the civilisations most connected with the expansion of our awareness as a species of the planets and stars were the Greeks and Romans, but Ancient Egyptians were also fascinated by the night sky and its mysteries. Celtic Reiki, was originated from a resonance between the trees and the Celtic connection to the trees as sacred entities. In its adaptation and evolution, it has grown to encompass great civilisations and their objects of spiritual and scientific growth.

The system of Celtic Reiki has come to encompass 5,000 years of philosophy, however, the foundations of our practice do not end there. For our exploration of our ancestry extends even further into the past, to a point where history and mythology blur into strange places that seem only to exist in the innermost reaches of our core perception; the prehistoric, lost civilisations of Atlantis and Lemuria.

The Mountain Range

The veracity of the existence of both Atlantis and Lemuria is widely debated and disputed to such an extent that it may hinder Celtic Reiki practice if a definitive attitude was adopted by me or the 'practice'. So, I prefer to leave the definition of these lost worlds to each Master or Practitioner to create individually and ask that they extend the same courtesy to their students.

In Celtic Reiki philosophy, we focus on the core dynamics of both Lemuria and Atlantis, (which are provided the concept of Mountain Range Realm) – a place of fire and thunder. The Mountain range extends from the high mountains at the north of the range, to the volcanoes of the south.

The peaks of the northern mountains are so massive that the entire realm can be viewed from the highest of these. This area of the Mountain Range, represents the observer, the viewpoint and the perspective from which all else is seen. The philosophy of the northern peaks is one of individual perception and the uniqueness that every observer has through their own senses and interpretation.

The fiery southern volcanoes personify the concept of adaptation, moulding and shaping of the world around us. For as all things are cleansed and reborn through fire, our perception can also be adapted through the shaping of energy, thought and connection. This Atlantean view of geometric shaping, combined with the perspective orientation of the Lemurian view provide Masters with an adaptability in their art unlike anything else available in energy therapies.

It is in the dynamic of observer-observed interaction that we comprehend the amazing principles of energy potential. The Celtic Reiki Master not only recognises the many essences of the different Realms, they also know that each can be viewed from an infinite array of perspectives and reshaped into forms as simple as a line, or as complex as the multi-faceted thought patterns of the genius mind.

The Mountain Range Realm is also where the harvesting and definition of essences takes place, as the Celtic Reiki Master orientates to the energy of trees, stones, the stars and the Earth. Once orientated, they adapt the parameters for their practice and create their own therapy of Celtic Reiki, with personal essences and a vast array of unique tools that are personally-defined.

The Furthest Ocean

The element of Water is emulated by the Realm of The Furthest Ocean and its endless depths of emotion, perception and cerebral creation. The oceanic realm is very different to that of the land; it holds secrets and mysteries beyond imagination and yet, the ocean is not the external place we believe it to be: it represents the internal world and the hidden knowledge we all possess at our very foundation.

The psychic abilities offered through the Furthest Ocean grant us access to intuition when treating, the ability of divination in Celtic Reiki readings and the empathy of higher cerebral abilities that give the impression of telepathy and a deep knowing of others' needs. Connection to the wisdom of old and the intelligences that exist beyond this point in time and space are gained by swimming in the ocean. Furthermore, by connecting to and working in the Ocean Realm, we glean information and knowledge that increases our sensitivity to any situation or circumstance.

THE FIVE MYSTICS OF CELTIC REIKI

An important element of Celtic Reiki Mastery is not only that essences and practice are affected by the 'place' or realm from which they are conducted, but also your perspective plays a huge part in the formation of a treatment or practice. As you work with the various essences, techniques, styles, and so on, you adopt a role, or what I call an avatar, that you use to hone and perfect the end results.

To illustrate this philosophy, imagine a group of people studying a piece of fine art. One of the group is interested in the aesthetic of the painting, whilst another is focussed on the artist that painted it. Another member of the group is fascinated by the history of the piece, one by its financial value. Each member of the group will perceive the work in a slightly different way, because of their perspective and the attitude they bring with their observation of the piece. The same could be said about the approach you take when working with Celtic Reiki.

Thus, the five Mystics of Celtic Reiki will help you

to alter the results you achieve, through the different roles you embody.

These five avatars are:

- The Alchemist
- The Wise One
- The Adventurer
- The Warrior
- The Master

Each Mystic has a unique perception of the world, the situation you're treating and the focus of the treatment, be it a client, a dynamic or you, yourself. For instance, a Warrior avatar will strengthen the effects of a treatment, acting as a custodian or guardian, enhancing the sturdiness of techniques and increasing the potency of essences used. Conversely, the same treatment conducted by a Wise One, will be looking at the insights that can be gained from the treatment, the knowledge of each essence used and how the techniques can yield further wisdom to assist the focus in their evolution.

Each Mystic is part of the Orientation and Calibration processes of a Celtic Reiki course, though the main viewpoint of each is discussed here for your reference.

The Adventurer

The first Mystic is that of the Adventurer, who, as the name suggests, is an explorer, a student, and a discoverer of uncharted territory. The purpose of enveloping the Adventurer avatar is to learn more about an essence, technique or practice in the Celtic Reiki experience. The Adventure is the very first Mystic that you encounter on a Celtic Reiki experience, for this Mystic helps you, not only to learn Celtic Reiki practice, but also to explore and discover new layers of wonder in the advancement of your therapy.

Whenever you embody the Adventurer Mystic, you automatically begin to experience treatments, essences, etc. at a deeper level of sensory perception. This denotes an increased awareness of how you are affected by any practice and a pushing of your current boundaries to glean 'more' from Celtic Reiki – more experience, more sensation, more awareness, more knowledge, and so on.

The Adventurer is bold, knowing their capacity to learn and explore. Whereas the Warrior is simply confident about their overall ability, the Adventurer's focus is in self-esteem and confidence that they can achieve greater ability. To the Adventurer, what some may call 'mistakes' are seen as opportunities and when a wrong-turn is taken, the Adventurer will learn as much as they can, so as to create change in the future and to develop a wise understanding of how the right, future path for each situation can be intuitively discovered.

The Mystic Adventurer permeates every level of Study, Practitionership and Mastery and is of particular use in the initial stages of Celtic Reiki development.

The Warrior

The embodiment of the Warrior Mystic is that of confidence in one's ability, determination and the knowledge that a person can do anything they set their mind to, providing they are willing to do what it takes to succeed. The Orientation to the Warrior avatar is usually conducted as part of the Practitionership stage and marks the ability of a Celtic Reiki Practitioner to have confidence in their ability, their methodology and their philosophical knowledge of their art.

As the Adventurer explores and discovers, the Warrior displays the courage to explore beyond the comfort zone, to innovate and have faith in what is discovered. The greatest strength any Practitioner or Master has, is belief in their own treasures. The Warrior Mystic also asserts the results they achieve, so when a client is resistant, because of scepticism or limiting belief, the Warrior will guide the client to transcend what is keeping them from expanding and assist in their personal growth.

It is common knowledge that no Celtic Reiki Master can make their client well, or manifest a goal on their client's behalf – for it is our job to act simply as a catalyst to the process. The client (or focus) must take on the responsibility for their own ability to heal, manifest, etc. for any practice to work, however, imagine a scenario where a car mechanic and a doctor give you a diagnosis for a headache; whose opinion would you trust and more importantly, who do you feel is more likely to help ease the headaches? This is the role of the Warrior, because by believing in yourself, you inspire others to believe in themselves also.

The Warrior is also an excellent avatar to employ when conducting Celtic Reiki readings, because this Mystic will increase the strength of the reading and connect at a greater level to sensory information. In turn this offers heightened clarity in visualisation and interpretation of the readings. Furthermore, the Warrior is the Mystic of psychic perception and encounters of the paranormal/otherworldly when working in a Celtic Reiki context, such as the incident with the Reflector (Demon), as recounted in Stories from the Sacred Grove.

The Wise One

The avatar of the Wise One is the healer and the keeper of secrets/wisdom. As one moves from the student and explorer phase of the Celtic Reiki training and through the elements of intuitive perception and building of confidence, the Practitioner enters a layer of practice that requires compassion, unconditional care and the ability to transcend one's own boundaries. Even in the Mastery of Celtic Reiki, the Wise One Mystic is an avatar that is revisited on a regular basis.

Treatments and practices that are conducted from the perspective of the Wise One take on a deep-acting quality that is centred on healing of past trauma and current challenges. The healer is also the contemplative; a profound being that gleans wisdom from every experience and learns from the situations they encounter. As you work, particularly in treatments, with the Wise One, you immerse yourself with the processes of the treatment and learn from them for future use. Knowledge and experience simply 'stick' with greater adhesion to the memory of this Mystic.

An integral part of the third Orientation, along with the Alchemist Mystic, the Wise One creates an ongoing and adaptive avatar that will be a steady companion on your Celtic Reiki path. If the Adventurer is seen as expansion and the Warrior is strengthening; the Wise One would be integration. The Alchemist conducts integration, in terms of the coalescence of two separate entities (a focussing and honing-in on a single goal or point). The Wise One is integration to create an all-encompassing, balanced, and evolving perspective. In visual terms we could imagine the Alchemist to be the eyes focussing in on a distant object, to clarify it, the Wise One is an acknowledgment of the peripheral vision to absorb as much of a scene as possible.

The Alchemist

By creating something new from two or more elements, the Alchemist Avatar favours the manifestation or creation of dreams in the physical world. The Magician and Spell Caster of the Celtic Reiki world, the Alchemist Mystic helps the Practitioner or Master to bring what is wished for into reality. Of course the attainment of goals is a process that transcends mere fancy – it requires planning and regular assertion, yet the dynamics created by the Alchemist inspire results that bring what is potential into reality.

Imagine wanting something so much (or not wanting it) that you think about that thing most of the time. Eventually, according to the magnetic laws of the Universe, you will bring that 'thing' towards you. Yet the mere dreaming and visualisation of that end result may create a meandering effect where the goal takes time to manifest or a dual-effect where ambiguous results are created. For instance, a person wants more time to spend with their family, so they manifest losing their job! The focussed, quantified results of the Alchemist dynamic, create a huge momentum and assist in the clarification surrounding manifestation and the goals a person requires.

Additionally, the Alchemist is excellent when used at the Master degree to harvest and create essences. Now, whilst the Warrior is often a better choice when working on the testing of essences, the Alchemist will enhance the definition of essences, honing in on results and effects. In many ways, Celtic Reiki essences rely a great deal on the parameters set by each individual Master, and this avatar not only helps create an arena for clear definition, but also hones every aspect of an essence into easily definable characteristics.

In other words, an essence applied using the Wise One Mystic may result in vague sensations or synaesthesia - "There was a slight pressure around this area of my head and some colours". The Alchemist Mystic's application is more likely to result in highly refined information – "There was pressure above my left eye, ascending to the crown and flashes of violet light".

The Master

The role of the Master Mystic is as the Mentoring and Teaching avatar, whose connection to Celtic Reiki overflows with integrity and the ability to instil that connection in others. The Master creates dynamics that are excellent for training others and the creation of learning environments, such as the Ki Classroom and Woodland Path.

Although, the role of the Master Mystic has a far broader range of influence than simply teaching, as they nurture an outlook of compassion and kindness, as well as strength of mind and spirit. A leader and guide to those who seek expansion and growth, the Master is connected to many secrets and sacred knowledge that can be accessed and imparted to inspire others with grace and power

THE FIVE LORES OF CELTIC REIKI

The five Lores of Celtic Reiki are not 'laws' to be obeyed as in modern society; they are guidelines, methodologies or ways of doing specific activities that can be viewed as a support framework for Celtic Reiki practice. Whilst the Lores are only made explicit in the very latest iterations of practice, they do offer the most wonderfully rich foundation, from which you can build a sturdy and effective method of practice.

Much has been said in connection to Celtic Reiki, both expansive and contractive. To define the 'Tao' of Celtic Reiki and to nurture the dynamics of expansive feedback, we use Lores, the first of which I weaved into the very fabric of the Celtic Reiki practices from their conception. Others have been introduced and many more will become appropriate in the future, though in this book, we shall ponder the main five. To best appreciate the nature of the Lores and how they affect our Mastery of Celtic Reiki, it would be helpful to have an understanding of how Celtic Reiki is perceived by others, both through presentation and assumption.

Most of the contractive feedback I've come across in connection to Celtic Reiki has been formed by those who have never actually had a Celtic Reiki Orientation/Attunement and can therefore be discounted. However, a minority of people who have experienced attunements and remain unimpressed have stated on occasion that Celtic Reiki "is not that different from Usui Reiki", which suggests, either the student has not focussed on their Celtic Reiki attunement (this is why we now have 'Calibration') or their Master did not conduct the attunement/was not actually a Master. In either case, the student's sub-conscious would simply adjust the conscious focus to what it knows to be 'Reiki' – in the ideals of Usui, as opposed to that of a Celtic Reiki perspective.

Reiki is a force, just as gravity is a force – we do not refer to bungee jumping or sky-diving as 'gravity', even though it is gravity that powers these activities. Yet, we do refer to the practices that require Reiki as a driving force as simply 'Reiki'. Can you imagine the confusion if people said "I'm doing a gravity for charity this afternoon!" or "Some people shouldn't do gravity for health reasons!" This is the bemusement I feel when I hear people talking of Reiki as the practice, not the force.

This may seem rather pedantic, however, when you have spent a third of your life originating and refining a practice and you meet with Usui Reiki Masters who say that Celtic Reiki is not 'real Reiki' or that Usui never visited Britain, it becomes relevant for all Celtic Reiki Masters to have a clear understanding that Celtic Reiki is not real Usui Reiki and that Usui has visited Britain – through the senses of every person in Britain that has studied Usui Reiki! Therefore, Celtic Reiki began as an adaptation of Usui Reiki practice and became a style of practice in its own right, just as a child grows up to become an independent adult that no longer needs to adhere to the education of their childhood teachers.

The attunement is vital in any form of Reiki practice (Orientation and Calibration as it is now known in Celtic

Reiki) because in the absence of an attunement, it is rather like a person bungee jumping without gravity—imagine somebody attempting to bungee jump from the ground! As soon as gravity is added it becomes a very different experience and this is why any Reiki practice cannot be learnt from a book. A qualified Master is required to act as a pilot, who flies the plane from which you sky-dive. A pilot cannot control gravity; she just knows the mechanisms needed to have an experience using gravity. The Master of any Reiki practice has parallel knowledge, when it comes to the force of Reiki; using the attunement (or similar) as a plane and their wisdom as a way of piloting the plane, they get you where you need to be to connect to Reiki and show how to style it from a particular perspective.

The confusion between the force and the practice has also made its way into Celtic Reiki, as I have noticed that people even dispute whether I created Celtic Reiki! My personal opinion is that I did not create Reiki, I did not create the Celtic philosophies, yet I did create a system called Celtic Reiki, which is my own perspective of Reiki (force) through a specific philosophy (Celtic originally and now expanded to encompass the beliefs of many indigenous cultures). The notion that a person can create a form of Reiki practice is imperative to all Masters, because if I can do it – you can do it. I do not dictate what Celtic Reiki is, I simply pass a baton with the intent that everybody who takes that baton will make Celtic Reiki their own, within the framework I originated.

This framework may be loose, yet it is very necessary, because it is important that an apprentice knows the foundations of Celtic Reiki and the rough map of the territory. There is not a single Usui Reiki Master in the world that teaches Reiki just as Mikao Usui did – his approach was unique, just as every person's perspective on life is unique. However, there are guidelines that mean a particular activity is encompassed by Usui Reiki practice and others are not.

My first Usui Reiki Master taught me to use 'Angel Cards' in my Usui Reiki practice – an element I incorporated with great success in the early days. These small cards gave people something to grasp in a subject that was beyond their 'comfort zone' at that point. In the early days of Usui Reiki practice in Britain, people did not usually know what to expect from a workshop, so the cards were a nice introduction to a magical, transformative day. Using Angel Cards is not Usui Reiki – but it is teaching methodology for some Masters and is therefore, acceptable. I once heard of Usui Reiki Master who used Tantric exercises as part of his Usui Reiki One training; a method that made everybody very uncomfortable in and out of his classroom! Now in a Tantric Reiki class, this would be acceptable, because attendees have an idea of what to expect, however, in Usui Reiki - no, it is not appropriate from my viewpoint.

As an example of why Lores are necessary, we could say that the Usui Symbols would not be appropriate in Celtic Reiki, just as the Ogham are not used in Usui Reiki. Conversely, the technique 'Reiji Ho' is used (either by name or under some other guise) and this provides Apprentices and Practitioners with a technique that helps them focus their practice, even though it was not derived from Celtic roots.

The five main Celtic Reiki Lores proffer a basic framework for learning, practice and teaching that explain some inherent methods and philosophies of Celtic Reiki methodology. To act within the definition of the Lores gives Masters and other users of the Celtic Reiki system peace of mind that they are offering others the practice with a spirit or viewpoint that is integrally 'Celtic Reiki', even though they have adapted and evolved the system. The Lores are not exclusive, but they do offer some precepts into the appropriateness of a particular way of acting.

One final important area of this debate is how, in any practice that can be adapted so widely, it is vital to maintain the attitude of choice and flexibility, as opposed to dogma and rigidity. For instance, I love the colour yellow, however I do not believe yellow is the 'best' colour or indeed the 'only' colour. I like chocolate – sorry, love chocolate! –

though I would not force others to eat it. A habit has formed in Reiki practices (as with many other practices) of taking the attitude of 'my way is the right way'. We create paths through the decisions we make and the actions we take – these paths are choices, not absolute 'law'. I would say that many people have a favourite colour and that it is good to eat food, however, beyond that it all boils down to personal preference.

No matter how Celtic Reiki is adapted or changed, I ask that each Celtic Reiki Master (and Masters of all Reiki methods) develop an attitude of differentiating personal choice from absolute law. To illustrate this, I originated Celtic Reiki with the concept of trees 'mimicking' Reiki as a form of treatment – as if it were the 'tree's perspective of Reiki'. Celtic Reiki has been adapted by others to being 'Reiki that flows from the Earth through our feet, instead of Universal energy from up above'. Now, you may be aware of my view of 'Reiki flowing' (I believe that Reiki exists beyond space and time, so it does not flow – it is our perception of it that creates the illusion of flow, rather like time or light through space), yet I would never say that this adaptation of Celtic Reiki philosophy is wrong – it is just another path.

When we examine the Lores, we see that Celtic Reiki embodies TreeLore, whilst Usui Reiki is often fixed in EarthLore and both have elements of EnergyLore and DarkLore. In recent years Usui Reiki has been focussed on 'getting back to the way it was originally done' and has thus become more focussed on EnergyLore, whereas I feel the original system, created by Usui, had a greater emphasis on DarkLore. I believe Celtic Reiki is most effective when used with a synchronisation of all five Lores – with a central Lore as the focus and the other four, concurrently and consistently positioned in the periphery of conscious awareness.

So, with this in mind, our initial exploration of the five Lores will offer a basic concept of how each Lore functions as part of the whole. However, the following synopses offer, but a brief taster of the complex, kaleidoscope of experience the Lores combine to create.

EarthLore

Let us begin our exploration of the Celtic Reiki Lores with that of the Earth. EarthLore is of the Earth in a physical sense and also with reference to the definition of our sensory and emotional experience of it. Earthlore also touches our conscious experience of all things, including spirituality and thought, which means that whilst our focus may lie with things beyond the physical world, we have a tendency to filter those things through the perception of our Earthly experience.

The force of Reiki is part of CosmicLore, however our intellectual estimation of Reiki and its use to power treatments, manifestation, etc. is of the EarthLore. Reiki undefined is CosmicLore, the act of treatment is TreeLore and the experience of Reiki within the context of that definition is EarthLore.

EarthLore represents the world and everything that is part of the world – it is the Earth and therefore it is the physical body. The body you believe yourself to be and the person you imagine I am are of the Earth and whilst, I believe, there is more that exists beyond the physical world, our ability to place parameters on the world around us and for it to parameterise us in return creates the world and is the core theme of EarthLore.

Therefore, EarthLore covers the methods and systems, the tools and techniques, and the principles and philosophies of Celtic Reiki. For example, the creation (in the sense of definition and application) of a Celtic Reiki Essence is EarthLore, as are the treatment methods used and the discernable results. The experience of an essence during treatment is not of EarthLore (this is TreeLore).

CosmicLore

CosmicLore exists beyond the world – it is of the stars; the intangible; the unknowable. When we look up at the night sky, we do not look through space, we look back through time, because we are not sensing what is, but what was. Always one step behind, our senses and Earthly experience is always of what was and never of what is. 'What is', is of the CosmicLore – the unknown and the undefined. As soon as you create parameters through TreeLore, so that CosmicLore can be grasped by the conscious mind, it is no longer of CosmicLore, but of EarthLore.

CosmicLore is a vital part of the Mastery, because it pertains to the existence of something beyond our comprehension. Celtic Reiki, for instance, exists in CosmicLore – always has, always will – however, during my experience with the Lone Tree (told in Stories of the Sacred Grove), I used TreeLore to create a reflection (definition) of Celtic Reiki in the EarthLore. At that moment, what you are now reading existed in the unknowable realms of CosmicLore, yet as each technique and philosophy was defined by myself or others, 'what is' becomes 'what was', like photographs of some fond memory.

CosmicLore is potential and also truth – the paradox is that as soon as we perceive it, it is no longer either and yet is remains both! Space and Time are both EarthLore, so when we define with those EarthLore parameters, we create more of the same, however the foundations (potential and truth) still exist in CosmicLore; they are simply negated in EarthLore, because of our integral grounding in the physical, defined world.

EnergyLore

EnergyLore is best described as what we perceive as the external existence, becoming the internal experience, or in more basic terms; the outside world flowing into you. Within the parameters of EarthLore, the Sun shines energy through space and in time to the Earth, where we experience it spatially and chronologically. The point is that sunlight does not travel anywhere; it simply exists in different states of being. In one state it is of the sun and in another state it is of your experience of the sun.

EnergyLore is therefore a dynamic that is present whenever what is 'outside' becomes what is 'inside'. The Orientation element of attunement to Celtic Reiki is EnergyLore, as is the cerebral and experiential learning of the practice. When you take what is without and make it what is within, this is the dynamic of EnergyLore in action. This book is EarthLore, the translation of the words in this book into your individual interpretation and the thoughts that stem from that interpretation are EnergyLore. This very personal and unique experience reaches deep into your perspective, creates change and growth and evolution and then it turns back on itself and becomes DarkLore.

DarkLore

If CosmicLore is of the Sun, then DarkLore can be compared with the Moon. Cosmologists believe that the Moon was created when the original Earth collided with another planet, known as Thea. The two planets impacted and converged to form the Earth and the Moon. Thus, when we look at the Moon (and with acknowledgement to the notion that we are all of the Earth), we perceive what was once internal, in the external world – or what was within, without!

The Moon is often viewed as mysterious and representative of what is hidden. DarkLore mirrors this inasmuch as it is our internal experience of everything we encounter, represented in an external form. What we do, how we act, the words we speak, write, and so on are all of the DarkLore. The Calibration processes of the Celtic Reiki attunement are DarkLore, as is the adaptation, use and teaching of our individualised forms of Celtic Reiki.

Hence, you might conclude that DarkLore is the reverse of EnergyLore, however, is the darkness really the opposite of light or is it the absence of light? Dark and Light have commonly been set up in opposition to each other, yet darkness is not a 'thing' in itself, it is the perceived lack of a 'thing'. The fascinating question that is derived from this philosophy is, does the 'outside world' exist as a thing within itself, or is it actually the perceived lack of a thing within itself?

TreeLore

The final place in our exploration of Celtic Reiki Lores is the TreeLore; the strength that binds all other Lores into our experience. There is a place where the observer (DarkLore) is connected to the observed (EnergyLore) and where what is known (EarthLore) meets that, which is unknown (CosmicLore). When we examine the symbol for infinity (∞), we see that the two loops converge at the middle to a single point and no matter how you travel along the path of the infinity, you will always pass this convergence at some point.

I often refer to trees as the place where the heavens meet the Earth, or the physical (leaves) meet the ethereal (sunlight). In this place, a frenetic dance occurs; a tango of energy as light and energy as the solid world. Trees, for me, represent this union of contrast; of abundance and lack; of light and dark; inner and outer; heaven and Earth. TreeLore is therefore the transformation of one dynamic or Lore into another. Trees symbolise birth, death and rebirth, the past, future and the present, as well as what is above, below and in between. They are the transitional point, where one thing can become something else and as such, TreeLore provides us with a system for change and transcendence.

This is the aspect of Celtic Reiki can be the most magnetic and powerful. For the blueprint or potential for Celtic Reiki exists in CosmicLore, the actual practice (method and philosophy) exists in EarthLore, yet in TreeLore, every person has the ability to make Celtic Reiki a unique celebration of their own perspective. At the place where outside meets inside, observer sees observed, learning becomes teaching, you and me are one, there exists TreeLore. And in TreeLore, all things converge into focus

KI ORIENTATION AND CALIBRATION

The most mysterious and profound cornerstone of any Reiki practice is the 'attunement'. This sacred process can be life-changing and transformative in unimaginable ways and has been for the millions of people who have studied some form of Reiki methodology. In a process that could be compared to the tuning of a radio to different broadcasts, the attunement connects the Apprentice to the force of Reiki and subsequently, enables them to interact with Reiki in a conscious way; focusing upon and directing different perspectives of Reiki with volition.

Originally titled 'empowerments' and what I now call the 'Orientation and Calibration' processes, attunements are an alternative way of teaching people how to work with Reiki and other facets of energy. Empowerments are very ancient practices, reported to have been used by mystics for many thousands of years. Having had many evolutions over time, the Orientation/Calibration method used in Celtic Reiki workshops is very different in routine to those used historically.

Energy Orientation and Calibration are still relatively mysterious processes, however the best way to describe what is happening is to imagine that you are speaking to somebody who had never seen the colour blue – how would you describe this to them in words so that they could understand what you mean? It is virtually impossible! However, if you could show them a piece of blue-coloured paper, they would instantly know what blue is and they would never forget it. This is the equivalent of an energy Orientation, which displays incredibly vibrant energy that may not have been experienced consciously before. The act of sensing energy (looking at the blue paper and recognising it consciously) is the Calibration part of the process.

I was trained in (Reiju) Empowerments and Usui Reiki attunements, which I adapted to encompass Celtic Reiki when I started to teach the therapy. I was not really comfortable with the term 'attunement', though, as it presupposed that I was 'doing' something 'to' the student. Every so often, I would also be confronted by a workshop attendee who explained that they noticed no sensory experience during the attunement. So I re-imagined the attunement in the form of the 'Energy Lesson', where I taught a lesson in energy for the student to learn. This simple repositioning of the terminology and explanation created a greater degree of success when teaching people how to connect to Reiki and other forms of energy/force.

Despite this shifting of description, the Energy Lesson was still not ideal, because it still placed so much emphasis on the teacher position. With the attunement, the Master 'did something to the student' and with the Energy Lesson, the Master 'taught something to the student'. It was this 'one-sidedness' that initiated the creation of the Orientation and Calibration process, which I now use exclusively on all my training events. The Orientation invites the apprentice to turn their attention to 'this point' (where the Reiki/energy can be sensed) and the Calibration is where the apprentice monitors their sensory data to decipher how they sense 'this point' to the fullest and most all-encompassing range of experience. This, not only balances the process equally between Master and Apprentice, it also assumes that the student will experience something, albeit to different degrees of sensitivity and with a wider variety of sensory feedback. It is hardly surprising that this methodology has extremely positive response and greater success than any of its predecessors.

When conscious awareness of Reiki is achieved via some form of attunement, it will never be forgotten and can always be used even if a Practitioner has not practised for many years. It does take a while to integrate fully with the physiological and cerebral systems, so that the various sensory effects and experiences increase with time, becoming stronger certainly over the three weeks after the Orientation. Of course, the more a person consciously practises the techniques and methods of Celtic Reiki, the better they understand it and the more results they will obtain.

Once an Orientation has been 'Calibrated', a range of sensory experiences become available to the apprentice and a period of profound exploration begins and evolves over time. This is the various Celtic Reiki Essences affecting the body and recognition of these effects supports the development of the Mastery skills. The reason one may experience these changes is due to the conscious focus adjusting to correlate and understand the information it is receiving from the senses that recognise Reiki (and other forms of vibrational energy).

So, until you learn to consciously recognise the subtleties in the Reiki at a direct, vibrational level, your brain translates Reiki as it would the data provided by your regularly used senses (Synaesthesia). Hence the effects seem to involve your sight, hearing, taste, smell and feeling.

Common effects include: Brightly coloured flashes of light, shapes and movement in front of the eyes, distortions, such as that caused by looking through heat, strobe effects, high pitched tones/tinnitus, rapid tapping inside the ear, as if a moth is flying about inside, inexplicable smells/perfumes that last only for a moment, peculiar tastes in your mouth, strange feelings of emotion, tingling, especially in the head, hands and feet, heat in hands, feet or head, pins and needles, trembling or spasms, imagery and 'random' thoughts, emotional outbursts, headaches or cold/flu-like symptoms, extremes of heat and cold, magnetic pulling/pushing in hands or body, vibrations/trembling sensations, especially in the spine, and the feeling of being touched or prodded.

These are just some of the sensory experiences you may find after a Celtic Reiki Orientation and Calibration; however, do not be surprised if you have other effects not mentioned here. These are all natural processes and are in no way detrimental to you. They will also ease and gradually disappear once you have integrated/learnt the elements of the Orientation – so do remember to cherish these effects, they are quite extraordinary and create very treasured memories.

My own training in Reiki empowerment and attunements varied in depth and description, yet it fascinated me to such an extent that I became passionate about the development, testing and application of different forms of teaching/learning experience involved with subtle energy and vibrational work. Over the years, this has evolved not only to spiritual endeavours, but also with regards to subjects as diverse as linguistics and social dynamics. With an expansion into new ways of teaching concepts and ideas, I have pioneered and experienced hundreds of Orientation styles, in addition to the ability to train others in altered states of awareness and advanced ability, simply by talking to them. I have devised new ways of 'broadcasting' Orientations at a distance, Self-Calibration to Reiki practices (et al), time-distorted and ongoing forms of Calibration where a person will attune upon activating some event (these are known as Click-Tracks or Triggers), and even Orientation and Calibration through reading text, such as this!

It is not only the style of Orientation that is important to keep in mind; it is also the nature of what is

Calibrated to. When I learnt Usui Reiki I was taught how to change the 'flavour' of Reiki for the purposes of physical or emotional treatment, for example. I was also taught how to connect to Reiki in different ways, for treatment across a distance or at different points in time, or to conduct Master practices such as attunements.

In Celtic Reiki, the traditions continue with the Orientation of essences (perspectives of ki), the Orientation of shape (the action and results of ki) and the Orientation to Energyscape or Ki-scape methods, which are complex dynamics of ki/energy that conduct a series of define results, based upon different criteria, etc. So, not only can you learn different essences, you can shape these to achieve different results and even build shapes and essences into a set of defined 'instructions' to create a multitude of effects.

Orientations and Calibration exist at every level of Celtic Reiki training and are often the most pleasurable and anticipated aspect of training. It is upon entering the Mastery of Celtic Reiki that these miraculous processes are the most relevant, because it is here that you learn how to conduct Orientations of different styles and how to teach others to Calibrate to them. What was once a profound experience for the apprentice, becomes a profound ability for the Master.

In modern varieties of Celtic Reiki training there are several Orientations for the apprentice to Calibrate towards. For example, in the Woodland Realm you have the various Celtic and Non-Celtic Tree Essences, the Elemental Essences and the Woodland (Elven) Essences. The Standing Stones has Orientations for the Nordic and Crystal Essences, whilst the Mountain Range covers 'methods' of working with Reiki, such as the harvesting of essences and the shaping of energy.

As the Master Orientates his Apprentices to the five Realms and all their contrasting and complementary essences and styles, the Avatars with their individual shaping abilities, and the Lores with their precise dynamics, a vast collection of practice abilities and techniques becomes available for Calibration. This rich and complex tapestry offers a diverse and simply extraordinary series of experiences to be had, not only at the time of Calibration, but for weeks, months, and years to come.

The Practitionership of Celtic Reiki

The very first experience I had of a Celtic Reiki Essence was that of Ailim. Harvested from a lightning-cloven Fir tree that offered me 'sight' once I had helped him to heal (see Stories from the Sacred Grove). After this particular experience, I made sure I always offer some form of treatment or energy work to a tree before harvesting an essence. It was my humanness that deceived me into thinking that the harvesting process was a matter of a 'trade'

During those early days, I decided that by offering some Reiki I could walk away with a new essence, yet whilst the Celtic Reiki system worked perfectly, my own sense of the essence was never as powerful or integral as it was that first time. The anthology of essences I 'collected' was special to me, I enjoyed the harvesting of new essences, but the process never offered as profound an experience as the Fir.

The reason, I now believe, for this situation is one of kindness or compassion. Physically, we take from nature, just as all other living things do – it is all part of the complex dance of life that takes place every day on Earth. The crux of the issue here is a philosophical one: To walk up to a tree, offer some form of Reiki treatment, then harvest an essence is the result of a transactional mentality. Offering treatment to a healthy, connected tree is rather like offering ice to an Inuit and as opposed to focusing on the individual tree, with his or her own perspective on life and unique desires, I saw a 'thing'; an 'it'.

Rather than harvesting an essence for incorporation into Celtic Reiki, by working with the trees and offering them what I saw as a 'fair trade', I began to realise that as a Celtic Reiki Practitioner and Master, my role was one of custodian to the natural world and as a guide who would help others view the natural world as I do, albeit from a slightly different perspective. One of the biggest surprises people comment on when I speak to them is how I refer to trees as living creatures and use 'him' or 'her', as opposed to 'it'. This comes from the innate care and respect I have for our tree friends – not only as a group, but as individuals. It was only when I started to walk my path, noticing and caring for all and every tree as a special being is that my connection to essences changed and I was, on several occasions, rewarded with an essence that was profound and fundamental to my being.

You see, if you work with the essence of a 'thing', it means very little. However, when you connect with another living creature and perceive a definitive personality, when you explore their distinctive and singular traits, as you learn about them, share experiences with them, spend time exploring each other, that 'thing' becomes a friend, a member of one's family – and we care about family and friends, much more than things. The essence of a loved one is an integral part of us – to chop down the thing in the garden for firewood is one perspective, to take a chainsaw to your best friend is a completely different matter. To feel love, kinship and connection to our tree friends, creates value in their essence and this is the goal of all Celtic Reiki users – to discover that overwhelming emotion that creates within us a deep care for all life.

When you do this, you do something very important; you create a rapport with plants as equals, not to dominate or take from, but as somebody who will offer assistance if required. Trees, on the whole, are not used to dealing with humans who act in this way and, once you have 'proved' yourself to the tree, they learn to trust, understanding that if just one person will see them as equal, then others can view them in that way too. By travelling through your life as a custodian, you transcend the transactional view, the fair trade, or the exchange and create a wonder and passion that is beyond Celtic Reiki – it is an essential, lost art that our Celtic ancestors knew, lived and breathed, because they existed at a time when human life appeared to be of little value in the wake of this huge, overwhelming force of the natural world. They needed to protect themselves from it, respect it and ensure that it was appeased. For the force of nature was a fickle and capricious entity, he could nurture or crush, she could offer life or take it away.

This was an age when the sacrifice of a human life, in all its fragility was nothing if it meant saving hundreds, by pleasing a deity and saving a crop of food. As we have evolved, we have arrived at a place where human life is sacrosanct above all else. We have mastered our environments and lifestyles to such an extent that we no longer need fear the natural world. Of course, we occasionally see its force and overwhelming power, but still we feel safe in our homes, cities and supermarkets.

Now I'm not saying that any of these things are negative – I, for one, adore shopping; at the supermarket or otherwise. Cities can be wonderfully vibrant places and I offer thanks every day for a roof over my head, security and warmth. The issue, as I perceive it, is that we need to create something new – a state of being that proffers kindness and stewardship to all living things. So, rather than simply using our evolved sensibilities to divorce ourselves from our inherent 'Earthliness' and then ignore the fact that we're only destroying ourselves when we destroy the natural world, we need to recognise that our evolution lies not with our power to destroy – it is with our power to nurture and protect.

In comparison to gaining the understanding of trees, the realm of humans is a much harder undertaking! The scientifically established fact that trees communicate with each other is not widely held as possible by the majority of people. The idea of trees communicating with humans is usually met with laughter and sarcastic comment. The thought of a person talking to trees is a concept that is mostly viewed as lunacy.

As a child I was thrilled and enchanted when I read the Lyall Watson's book 'Supernature', in which the author describes the reaction of plants to a person who was intending to do them harm, by burning their leaves. If a plant can produce a physiological reaction to the intentions of a human being, then a human being can have a physiological reaction to intentions of a plant. If you understand this reaction in yourself, you can interpret it into a complex form of communication and develop a way of conversing.

Once you have reconciled this concept with yourself, you may find resistance from family, friends and other people you come into contact with. To create a commonly held belief of how the natural world can be viewed through different eyes will happen in time, although within yourself you can realise that the views of others do not matter that much if you do not want them to. People who try the practice of 'tree hugging' may feel very self-conscious at first but, with practice they find the experience such a profound one that they do not care how 'silly' they look in the eyes of others.

It would be unfair of me to place the immense task of reinventing one's views towards trees (and indeed the Earth) on the shoulders of a Celtic Reiki Apprentice without some advice of where to start. So, if you have just Calibrated to your first Orientations or are new to the practice of Celtic Reiki, the best starting place is to increase your familiarity to the essences through systematic practice. If you feel the need, work with the Ogham to increase your awareness of the vibrations triggered by each, understand the practical applications of these, and work with the concept of treatment forests. When you feel confident that you have mastered these objectives, set aside a period of time each week to interact with nature. Maybe by travelling to a forest or moorland, your local park or your garden and if these are not feasible, try connecting at a distance.

Your first steps in creating your individual practice of Celtic Reiki may be to offer treatment to a sick plant, or some strengthening Reiki to a tree that is weak, spindly and tossed about by the wind. You may wish to work on more physical levels, by fertilising the soil with plant food or by joining a local preservation society. Your work can be completely energetic such as connection to Reiki for the protection of the rainforests or to nurture the new plants of spring. Do not wait for encouragement or provocation, just follow your intuition and do whatever you can, whatever feels right.

Get into the habit of doing something for nature every time you use Celtic Reiki for yourself. For example, if you perform a paid treatment for somebody, you might send some distance healing energy to the trees whose essences you used in the treatment, or save some of the money and put it towards the cost of planting a tree locally.

When you are manifesting a goal with Celtic Reiki, plant an acorn or Yew berry in the ground (making sure you are not infringing any laws and remembering that all parts of the Yew tree are poisonous!) If you assert yourself with Celtic Reiki, you could make a donation to a charity that works with nature, or write a letter to your local politician to help protect your local environment.

If you use Celtic Reiki to resolve an issue or problem in your life, remember to recycle your bottles, use less water in your bath that day or go out and treat a tree for five minutes. This is not an exchange, because, by returning a favour you are increasing the bond between you and the Earth; gradually these individual and isolated acts of kindness will spill out and merge into a perspective of compassion and care for the world around you. This, in turn, will create a superior relationship with the essences and enhance your intuitive, connective and sensory abilities.

As you give to the Earth and all creatures, so you will receive improved talents when working at source with the trees and plants used in this system of Reiki practice. Eventually this will evolve into the capacity to communicate with trees and work with them directly in fine-tuning your sensory and Reiki-connection abilities. The trees may show you variations on essences to achieve different results or a perspective better matched to your individual abilities. They may help you boost your connection, or give something far beyond your expectations.

When you reach this stage of your learning, there are two things to bear in mind. Firstly you should never expect recompense from your efforts in helping nature; this is not about exchange it is about your integrity and role as custodian. Give to the trees and to nature freely – you will have your own sense of achievement as thanks for your effort.

Secondly, always remember that some trees will not trust you, especially in areas where they have been abused. Humanankind is adept at producing much wonder and much terror and it is a part of the human condition that we impose ourselves upon all other things, including each other! This is something that I was aware of when originating Celtic Reiki and I have attempted to readdress in more recent work with nature.

The Essences of Celtic Reiki Practice

As in many other forms of Reiki practice, we can use some form of 'trigger' or 'statement of intent' to alter the specific perspective of ki or 'essences' we require in a treatment or manifestation environment. The idea of sacred sounds or symbols being used to trigger a particular force or flavour of energy was one favoured by Mikao Usui, originator of the Usui Reiki system. He devised a method where a student could learn the connection to Reiki through Reiju Empowerment. Then a collection of sacred sounds (Kotodama) were used as mantras to help the student decipher contrasting layers of Reiki for different purposes. Later, Usui used sacred symbols that the student drew with a finger or visualised to create this differentiation.

The devices did not hold power within themselves, it was an association made during or just after the empowerment that embedded the students' use of the symbols and mantras. Layers of Reiki explored in the empowerment were later reactivated by the Master when demonstrating the symbol or Kotodama. This forms unconscious connections for the student, who can then produce the same triggering results as the Master, although their sensory feedback will often differ slightly. As an alternative way of conceptualising this process, think about the reaction we have to certain words and how they trigger an emotional, cerebral, or even physiological response.

In the origination of Celtic Reiki I used characters from (or based upon) the Ogham or Celtic alphabet. Thus, when learning to use the system, students have, in many instances, a symbol and corresponding mantra for each essence (each and every essence has a phrase or mantra that can be used to trigger that particular essence). This offers the student various tools to work with until they feel comfortable with connecting to the essences directly.

A very important distinction that has been misinterpreted by some is that between the Ogham, when used without Orientation and Calibration to Celtic Reiki, and the effects afterwards. The Ogham has been around for centuries and comes with its own associations and 'energy' – if a person works with the Ogham, they are not working with Celtic Reiki unless they have Calibrated to do so. I have seen people suggesting that Celtic Reiki can be practicsd by simply using the Ogham – this is not the case, for whilst energy can be triggered by the Ogham, it is not the energy that is recognised as Celtic Reiki and is, thus, misleading to prospective apprentices or clients when used in this way.

Harmonics and Pure Essences

A fascinating concept, which is rarely encountered in energy therapies, but does play a substantial part in that of Celtic Reiki, is the idea of 'harmonics'. The harmonics of an Essence are the 'extra' perspectives encompassed within the essence, other than those of the original tree.

So the tree that acts as a source for the essence of its species will not only tell of its own perspective, it will offer the perspective of its species and on occasion its woodland or forest. Thus a Rowan tree in an Oak dominated forest may have a Duir-orientated perspective of Luis. This Duir-tinged view of the Luis essence is an harmonic.

An actual example of harmonics from the essence of Ioho, which was harvested from several Yew trees. Each presented an individual perspective as part of the Ioho Essence. Although if you strip away the individuality of the trees, you will find a 'pure essence' – this is the perspective of the species 'Yew' as opposed to several individual trees. The pure essence will be the same no matter how many trees you harvest the energy from because it is the essence of 'Ioho'.

This means that when you use the essence of the trees, you are connecting to the perspective of an individual tree or possibly many trees. However there is a way of stripping down the vibrations of an essence to gradually negate the individual views and perceptions of the source trees if you want to: the essence of each species of tree you require.

As you work with the stripping technique to hone in on a pure essence, (and therefore removing the individual traits for that particular application), the effect, I perceive, is akin to stripping white light into its constituent colours. Thus you achieve a change in the frequency of the essence and create different results in its application.. I have tended to find the overall consequence here is that the unaltered essence is more physical whereas the lighter, purer essence is more spiritual. The original essence works within minutes or hours, whereas the pure essence may take weeks to show signs of effect, however these effects will also have a deeper action.

So, depending on the holistic layers you wish to work on, you would strip as much or as little as you feel necessary for a particular client or situation. This enables you to achieve a much wider variety of results from a single essence and over time you will be able to strip the harmonics from each essence to a very precise layer of perspective. This in turn, will achieve very specific results

Stripping the Harmonics

Connect to the essence you require and feel it in your head, your hands and your arms. Now close your eyes and visualise a wall of light emanating from you. Now imagine this light getting 'thinner' in width – not lessening the strength of the energy, but reducing the actual 'thickness' of the wall.

When you feel this reach a single line, you have reached the 'Emotional/Cerebral Level. Expand the light again, keeping the sensation created by the vibration the same. To go to a spiritual level, repeat the exercise again and upon reaching a single line, you will have achieved this. You can do this one more time to reach the pure essence and this will work very deeply on you and your client, altering deeply rooted trauma, etc.

An Essence for Each Season

A popular technique among Practitioners pertains to the calendar. This method is very much down to 'taste' and will depend on your personal viewpoint as to its effectiveness. However in simple terms – the Evergreen trees are more potent in winter, the Deciduous trees in summer and the emphasis changes in each essence throughout the year – the cycle of Ruis, for example, is more relevant to 'preparation for change' in spring, and the 'accepting of change' in autumn.

You will also find that at some times, particular essences are stronger overall than at other times of year – this is because their resonance is in accordance with your resonance. Make notes of these shifts in a diary and you will soon see a pattern emerge. Use this to find your preferred essences for use at their most potent times of year. There should be one, possibly several essences per month – use these (at peak times) as much as possible on yourself and on others for even better results.

Some Masters believe the season is irrelevant to the potency of an essence, because it is winter (or summer, spring, autumn) somewhere on the Earth throughout the year. My personal view is yes, it is always winter from an Earth-wide perspective, however, is it winter all year round from your physical viewpoint (as opposed to your intellectual perspective)? The answer is to make notes about your particular sensations with particular essences at different times of year, as this will display what is the best approach for you as an individual.

THE FOUNDATION TREATMENTS

Selestrhy and Fwddiau

Two of the basic cornerstones of Celtic Reiki therapeutic practice are Selestrhy (Sell-less-tr-hee) and Fwddiau (Vowed-thee-eye): The Heavens and the Void. These two 'scanning' and treatment styles focus on the intuitive application of Celtic Reiki and the enhancement of sensitivity to vibrational change. In other words, use of Selestrhy creates intuitive or psychic awareness and Fwddiau will help you to distinguish different essences, vibrational issues, etc. Practice of these techniques can lead to some amazing sensory abilities, such as the ability to know future events in connection to your clients and the effect of 'seeing' your client's dis-eases, just by looking at them.

These easy to use, yet incredibly powerful techniques are so varied in results and potent in effect that together; they form the foundation of Karmic Regression Therapy (Karmic Reiki). Adapted for use with Celtic Reiki practice, they offer much of the same feedback with intuitive readings of a client's physical health, emotional and cerebral wellbeing, ancestral trauma and even displaying prophetic ability with relation to your client's future. Yet it is within the valuable use with essences and shaping skills that Selestrhy and Fwddiau come into their own, helping the Practitioner to master the different essences in preparation for teaching and harvesting.

Selestrhy – The Heavens

Beginning with Selestrhy, which embodies the shifting of the Heavens, the fluidity of the air and all the potential of the Universe, the hands (and eventually the mental focus) of the Practitioner are used to sense the dynamic patterns of the client's bioenergetic field. Resembling a graceful dance, the Celtic Reiki Practitioner is guided to work at various points, where gentle stroking, energetic swirling, dynamic pulsing and balletic finger movements take place. Without volition or conscious intervention, the Practitioner can concentrate on the myriad joys of internal sensation and imagery as they relax and let their intuitive, subconscious perform of powerful treatment. Often accompanied with a brilliant 'light show' of shapes and coloured light, this remarkable technique is one of the simplest to conduct.

Technique:

To conduct a Selestrhy treatment, simply start with a connection to your client by placing your hands either side of their head, about an inch or two away from their temples (without touching their head). There will be an internal shift of sensation, after which, state in your mind that you are going to treat your subject with Selestrhy.

When you feel a good connection to Celtic Reiki (with or without triggering named essences), move to the side of your subject and place your hands over their abdominal region. Continue to nurture your connection to Reiki until your hands begin to move to a new position; this will feel like a magnetic pull or push and can be disconcerting at first, but just allow this to happen. It is important not to make a change happen, or resist the movement when it does – just go with the flow!

If your hands move to their fullest extent, feel free to travel around your subject to obtain a more comfortable position for yourself. Remain at each position until your hands once again move of their own accord. At the end of the treatment, go to your subject's head area and finish with a final head connection.

Fwddiau – The Void

Fwddiau is the Void, although rather than a complete non-existence of anything, the Void in Celtic Reiki is a lack of vibrational potency or some form of distortion. These form a void in certain areas of the wellbeing of a client. Healing the Void, through scanning, sensing and treatment (of affected dynamics) promotes health for your client and a heightened degree of sensitivity in your energy-awareness abilities.

The Void effects that are sensed by Fwddiau are a wide range of sensations that will affect your hands, arms and other parts of your body, internally and even 'around' your body. These effects can be heat, icy cold, itching, formication (the sensation of insects crawling across the skin), spasms/twitching muscles, stabbing, tickling, breezes, and many other unusual feelings. Each of these represents a different type of distortion in your client's bioenergetic field and can be related to some physical or emotional dis-ease.

As you scan for Void effects, you will discover how to recognise these through sight, sound, taste and smell, as well as at a direct, vibrational level. Upon clearing the effects, you heal the associated dis-ease they are connected to.

Technique:

To conduct a treatment using Fwddiau, simply start by connecting to Celtic Reiki via a 'head connection': place your hands either side of your subject's head and feel an internal shifting, as with Selestrhy. Then use your non-dominant hand to 'scan' your subject's body, sensing the Void sensations in the aura/bioenergetic field surrounding the body. Upon discovering a Void effect, focus Celtic Reiki essences of your choosing at the location until the Void has ceased or 10 minutes have passed.

Upon clearing the Void, repeat the scanning until you have located and cleared as many effects as possible in the treatment time. Complete the treatment with a final head connection and then bring your subject back into the room.

A FOREST OF ENERGY

Celtic Reiki essences can be applied in a combined form to create new essences; the vibrations of the various tree essences form a 'forest of energy' or 'Treatment Forest'—each unique in its own right.

The letters of the Celtic Ogham (alphabet) construct words that can to write a 'book' of treatments and symptom cures. The combination of essences (tree perspectives) in a Treatment Forest works on many levels, changing a person in a multitude of ways; empowering them to alter their path and discover their unique place in the universe. This adaptability makes a combination of Celtic Reiki essences very powerful. Energy, wisdom and life combine in an amazing synthesis.

The process of 'writing treatments' differs from triggering an essence through the use of a symbol, treating with this essence, and then changing the essence – here you use the single essences one after the other. When you write a treatment in the form of a Forest of Energy, you define a refined and specific perspective of energy that can be used across a whole treatment, resonating more strongly and acting on deeper layers of being.

A simple example of writing a Celtic Reiki Treatment Forest is for somebody who has lost their way in life, they cannot see a way forward and look only to the near future – trying to find the benefits in a short-term answer rather than seeing the long-term conclusions. This evolves into a situation where their perpetual thinking causes an inability to do anything and they become paralysed by fear of doing the 'wrong thing'. The sentence here could be:

- Finding the way through the labyrinth: Gort
- Seeing the bigger picture: Ailim
- Clearing mental confusion: Huathe
- Finding personal truth: Uilleand
- Creating a sanctuary: Koad
- Creating stillness: Mor
- Increasing the power of the treatment: Ioho

So you would begin a treatment in your preferred way, perhaps with a request for assistance from unseen friends, deep breathing, or some light meditation. Then draw the Ogham sentence on your palms, over the client, or just visualise - GAHUKMI. Now complete the entire treatment by working with hand positions, intuition or with Selestrhy – occasionally reasserting the Ogham symbols if you feel this is necessary.

As you practise with the symbols or purely through sensory feedback, the essences become fixed in your body's 'muscle memory' and intuitive knowledge. Hence, you will be able to create treatments of more elaborate complexity – at first, intuitive guidance will help you, then over time you will be able to consciously use the essences with volition to perform potent, effective treatments. Remember to draw the symbols as a word in one fluid process – not in bits-and-bobs throughout the treatment, as this may act to create a confused definition and become too fragmented

The Treatment Forest & The Woodhenge

As we have explored previously, all treatments, routines, and methods in Celtic Reiki are derived from definition. The style in which a practice is defined will form the basis for its effectiveness and the results achieved. The more clarity you can instil with the parameters of a treatment, the greater the results.

Whenever you conduct a treatment, you are often wise to limit the number of vibrations you use at any one time, as using many different essences can cause your definition to become fragmented. This will make a treatment seem 'bitty' and without a solid, definitive focus. To avoid this happening, the Treatment Forest can be used to plant essences into a clearly defined 'set' of intents and create a forest (Stone Circle, etc.) that can be used as a single essence, thus replacing many.

The concept of a Treatment Forest is very useful, especially when treating people who require many different essences to assist in easing their various situations and diseases. Yet the forest is always different, because each, individual tree lends itself to a whole and the autonomous forest has many unique dynamics and changes. Next time you walk through a wood, try to sense the energy of the woodland as a whole and then communicate with the individual trees and see the difference – although each tree is part of the whole, the forest is a complete contrast; greater than a combination of single trees.

Consequently, how do you use many different essences in a treatment, keeping a strong intent and focus, yet maintaining the integrity of each individual tree essence? For the answer to this, we look to another form of therapy and the personal development system known as The Viridian Method. In the methodology of VM is a technique known as Parallel Projection, which is translated for Celtic Reiki practice to the Woodhenge (or Stonehenge, if working within the Standing Stones Realm).

The Woodhenge is the technique by which Woodland Realm essences can be stacked into a single treatment essence, yet maintain all of the original qualities. This works on the basis that each single essence is defined in the same place, at the same time, yet in different layers of perception.

To grasp this, imagine that you walk through a forest, taking a path that leads you past many different trees. At various points along the path you stop and interact with an individual tree. Now in your linear perspective, you experience this journey as 'one tree after another', however if you step outside of time, all the interactions occur without a time distinction. In other words, it is like reading a book – all the events exist in the book, though the linear journey of reading the book is necessary for you to become consciously aware of those events!

The creation of the Woodhenge is where you simply define a set of parameters with a specific structure. In energetic terms, you split your client throughout several realities, treat them with a single essence in each reality and them 'put them back together' in this reality.

Without getting too technical, this process is based upon a parallel with the principle of 'Photon Duality'; a concept in Quantum philosophy. This is where a particle of light (Photon) can exist in two different places at the same time if it possible for it to do so. If you create more possible paths for the photon to travel along, it will do this also – all at the same time! It truly is possible for the photon to be in two places at once!

Of course the process is much simpler in practice than it may sound here, because you only need define a treatment as "The Woodhenge" and then activate each essence you wish to add to the treatment.

Once you have done this, simply continue with the treatment style you have chosen as you would normally. The thing to remember is that you can place several (all, if you wish) treatment essences into a single Woodhenge and treat your subject for a whole hour – every time you add an essence, they will be technically receiving their hour treatment, multiplied by the number of essences! So if you use five essences in a Woodhenge treatment, you are offering your client five hours of treatment in just one hour of time!

BEYOND THE WOODLAND REALM

A s you move beyond the Woodland Realm of Celtic Reiki practice, you find connection to other forms essences, such as the Runic and Crystal Essences of the Standing Stones Realm, plus the Stellar and Stargate Essences of the Celestial Realm. As with the Tree Essences, the Runic Essences can be used in divinatory 'Oracle Readings' for clients (see the following chapter). However, an amazing form of treatment for clients and you, in the form of a self-treatment, are those using the trinity of Stargate, Crystal and Stellar Essences to create a rich, sensory experience on higher layers of consciousness.

Here you use the Stargate Essence to create a connection or synthesis between the Earth (Crystal Essences) and the stars (Stellar Essences); expanding your solid world consciousness into the ethereal realms of spiritual experience, where you can meet and interact with forms of higher consciousness and intelligence. The process is studied in depth during your Celtic Reiki training and can only be achieved to full effect, after you have Calibrated to the appropriate Orientation, though it is listed here for your interest.

Stargate Trinity Treatment Technique:

1. Lay your client on the treatment couch, or sit them in a padded chair, ensuring that they are comfortable. If you are conducting a self-treatment, simply sit in a chair or lay down with your open palms on your body.

2. Close your eyes and make a head connection by placing you hands either side of your client's temples – near the skin, but without touching.

3. Activate the first essence, which will be a Crystal Essence of your choosing. Your hands can remain at the same position throughout the treatment, or you can move them as you intuit.

4. Maintain this connection for 3-5 minutes before triggering the Stargate Essence and continue to hold this perspective for a further 3-5 minutes.

5. Now activate the third and final trigger, which will be your chosen Stellar Essence. At this point you may wish to guide your client through a meditation, or, if self-treating, use visual imagery to heighten your experience. Continue at the level of these three essences for the duration of the treatment.

6. Once you have conducted the treatment for the desired time, bring your client back into the room and offer them some water to drink.

7. Ensure they are fully aware and comfortable before asking them to stand up.

The Transcendent Practitioner

Shifting, Shaping and Going Beyond

Once you have worked alongside your Celtic Reiki Master, through the basic Practitioner treatments, you will be asked to begin your advanced training. This will incorporate your psychic awareness abilities and your shaping of Ki skills. All forms of energy, including Ki/ Reiki exist both as vibration (type/flavour/essence) and as dynamic (honed result/action/shape). Reiki practices often focus on the type of Reiki used for various results, such as physical treatments or emotional issues. In Celtic Reiki we also take into consideration the dynamic or shape of Reiki.

Imagine you are painting a picture using different colours (vibrations) of paint. Each colour or mixture of colours will produce a different end result, however, when you combine these colours with shapes (dynamics) you can create finely crafted and accurate results. The employment of shapes not only adds definition to the painting, it also required the colours be used to particular effect, therefore giving greater meaning and purpose to the application of each colour. This is analogous to how we shape the essences of Celtic Reiki to achieve precise results.

The Universe is energy. Energy that cannot be created, or destroyed – only changed from one form to another. This is the basis of many belief systems, over thousands of years of human culture and over many different continents. We have learned this concept in many different ways and through an endless variety of methods. As we have reached each level of understanding, our awareness of energy has expanded and necessitated fluidity in our perception akin to that of the energy itself.

The connection to and experience of 'Universal Energy' is increasingly popular in methods such as Reiki practice and numerous other techniques. Many of these systems observe a two-dimensional approach to energy: a basic journey from one place to another. This creates a passage through states of being, so for example, energy can be employed in healing to travel from a state of dis-ease to a state of health, in manifestation from not having something, to having it, and in meditation from being conscious, to being aware of other layers of existence, etc.

In recent years, the transitions have become more sophisticated as we adapted our perception to shift and shape energy beyond a simple two-point reasoning (straight line) – creating spirals to expand and intensify energy vibrations, triangles to form a journey via a secondary point, or a square to arrive at a destination via two opposing points. Using the example of an energy triangle, energy is focussed from one point (You), to a second point (problem), to create a third point (solution) and this returns to you - the first point. This is not to say that energy 'travelled' along this path, only that the dynamic created in energy was that of a triangle (the energy acts as a triangle; affecting three points of focus). Using techniques such as this, our knowledge and facilitation of energy has been increasingly elaborate and we have grown in knowledge and awareness as a result of this.

This process of development enabled us to be consciously aware of higher and higher vibrations of energy, jumping up the range of frequencies and rekindling awareness of our previously ignored (consciously) energy systems (Peri-systems), in turn awakening from our energetic naivety to a place of enlightenment, both spiritually and technologically.

In the past few years, the shaping has expanded to embrace an even wider range of ability and complexity with the application of secondary forms, in a three-dimensional method of dynamic. Geometric shaping in the form of tetrahedra, spheres, cubes and pyramids, meant a period of rapid progression and exponential learning existed in energy therapies and arts. Results not only became more defined, but the chance of success also increased as many different aspects of a person could be included in a single treatment, hence tackling many challenges in one carefully planned session.

Further dimensions to the definition of energy shifting reached a level where the old point-to-point view of a path was actually negated! No more did a client have to travel from dis-ease to health – it could be instantaneously achieved through as little as a single treatment and this was absolutely miraculous to behold. Working towards a goal, or going from one state to another; the approach we have been accustomed to, in the 'linear view of energy', means that we are moving away from our intended destination as we move towards it. The path between A and B can be used in reverse to regress and devolve if other factors in the holistic nature of a person are inclined to.

The notion of a four-dimensional shape (which our three-dimensional minds can only be 'aware' of as opposed to actually visualising) offers us the scope to move beyond the linear, path approach.

When used to full potential the shaping of energy can perform many interesting and amazing tasks, as we access energy perspectives that are usually unknown to us. The integration of this approach into Celtic Reiki from the

Viridian Method, etc. has offered another level of effectiveness to all the different intents we can achieve within the system.

By taking the principles of 'shaping Reiki', we can create a result similar to stepping out of physical reality, doing what we need to do and then stepping back in with new vibrational patterns. This realigns us to new paths, allows us to create multiple paths, or even negates the need for a path altogether!

Exercises

These exercises have the prerequisite of some form of attunement or Calibration to a Celtic Reiki Orientation. If you have experienced an Usui Reiki attunement, or some other form of empowerment, you will be able to work well with the following techniques.

In order to maximise your success with these exercises, ensure that you work with each one in order and then only move on after you feel completely comfortable.

Exercise One – Line or Spiral

In this simple exercise, stand in front of a person or object and visualise yourself directing a beam of Reiki/energy/light at it. You can use your hands if it focuses your intent, or just 'beam' it at the object.

Once you have done this, attempt to beam energy in a straight line at an imaginary object, or distant place/event.

If you wish, you can try 'spiralling' the energy outwards from you at the centre to the outermost point of the spiral, the object (this intensifies the resulting dynamic). An interesting version of this is to imagine energy spiralling in at you and see the effect!

Exercise Two – Triangle

This exercise works with a challenge or issue that you have in your life currently. Stand in an open space and imagine the problem diagonally to your right. Imagine that you are beaming Reiki or light at it, as you did with Exercise One. See the energy burst through the problem and turn to the left, where it starts to create a solution. Then bring this solution to you, diagonally from the left hand side.

Exercise Three – Square

For this exercise, you can use a desired goal that is either blocked by two conflicting issues (challenges), or two imagined objects (such as pillars or even people). The goal could be, for example, that you want to write a book, although your job does not allow you the time - if you leave your job, you will not have enough money to support yourself.

Visualise the two challenges, or objects on each diagonal to you, and then imagine you are directing Reiki/ light at them simultaneously. Watch the energy work through the two points and then converge on a point opposite you to form a square. If you wish, you can then imagine yourself at the opposite point, soaking up the energy of your goal.

Exercise Four – Cube

This exercise is a little more complex and involves multiple 'targets', so for ease of learning, you can imagine three people; two diagonally from you, and one diagonally from them – opposite you. You want to 'beam' Reiki at the person in front of you, but cannot, so imagine two streams of energy coming from your feet and beam these either side of you, to the 'diagonal people'. Then produce similar streams at head level and see all four beams working through the two people. The energy intensifies and is then directed at the focus person opposite you.

With practice, you will be able to substitute the two diagonally positioned people for up to 4 conflicting issues and then see a single solution opposite. When you feel that the Reiki or light has reached the solution, see yourself standing in the opposite position 'soaking up the energy'. If you are finding that the problems are overwhelming you, you can then visualise yourself in the centre of the cube, unaffected by the challenges.

CELTIC REIKI AND THE PSYCHIC SENSES

When working with the Oceanic Realm of Celtic Reiki (The Furthest Ocean) you can greatly enhance your prophetic, intuitive and psychic abilities. Add to this, practise with essences from the Standing Stones and Celestial Realms, along with essences such as Saille, Luis, Duir, etc., and you will find that your vibrational senses light up with activity. Your ability to read, decipher and interpret this information will also improve dramatically. Furthermore, if you're interested in developing your psychic abilities, I would recommend looking into vReiki training (for the Jiki elements) and reading my book vPsychic (mPowr Publishing).

When using your psychic abilities, your main 'tool' is your body, emotions and mind. The way in which you interact with any given environment or practice will dictate how much information you receive as well as the clarity and accuracy of that information. Therefore, the key to psychic training using Celtic Reiki is regular exercise you use in your everyday life which will help you develop your body and mind's natural abilities to sense what is usually hidden and beyond the realms of perception. The areas of focus when working with Celtic Reiki and the aspects of you that respond to psychic development training are:

- Clearing and Healing
- Raised Awareness and Focus
- Increased Sensitivity
- Intuitive Ability
- Imagination and Descriptive Skills
- Assertion and Confidence

Once you have started to develop your psychic practices in the Oceanic Realm, you will find that a whole range of new and exciting activities are available to you, such as:

- Guide Work
- Communication with Nature Spirits, Ghosts, and other Entities
- Lost Soul Work
- Intuition and 'ESP'
- Psychometrics
- Personal Readings
- Karmic Regression and Past Life Readings

Developing your sensory skills in order to understand the subtle information embedded within your energy senses and perceiving other levels of being can be an exciting and rewarding exercise, yet, as with any Reiki-based healing practice, psychic development also requires regular practice and a commitment to evolve as a person in many ways. Whilst some people do retain varying degrees of psychic ability from childhood, most of us have to relearn how to use our additional sensory abilities.

Psychic ability is not really about 'seeing ghosts', although this is very often the aspect of it that catches the imagination. Psychic ability is about developing your senses to perceive the world around you in a different way; whether that is working with the subtle information contained in the environment or objects, helping people with therapeutic Reiki treatments, personal readings and past life information or sensing beings that do not have physical form. If working with Celtic Reiki in the other Realms is about healing, self-mastery and enlightenment, in the Oceanic Realm practices are sensory, communicative and intuitive.

Very often, the first step in evolving your psychic senses is to leave behind any preconceived ideas about what you think is going to happen and practising techniques that sometimes appear to bear no relation to the end result! In fact, psychic training can be compared to Operatic Performers developing the ability to sing, they do not sing for long periods in favour of breathing exercises and abdominal crunches!

The initial stage of the Oceanic Realm training process is integral to evolving yourself to the required level of sensory health. If you have had major trauma or emotional upheaval in your past, this may hinder the ability to raise your vibrations. Therefore it can be challenging to focus on the subtle senses and receive the information contained within its dynamics. The heavy vibrations of fear, anger, grief, hatred, jealousy and so on, all hinder psychic abilities.

Therapeutic treatments are an excellent way of assisting this process and this is often why Celtic Reiki Masters report enhanced psychic and intuitive abilities.

The initial stages of your psychic enhancement may present you with vague mental images, words, coloured light, faint smells or tastes, strange and indescribable feelings. These are all signs of the initial awakening within you as your conscious brain attempts to decipher all of this new information it is recognising.

How you sense the data from your energy senses depends on how you 'work' as a person and, because we all work in a unique way, this means discovering what your dominant synaesthetic associations are and how these affect your experience. Some people have a visual experience while others hear more. You may be a person who feels things or even works with smells and tastes. The sensory experiences you have are not actual sense data, but the synaesthesia associated with your energy or subtle senses (Peri- Systems). Once you know what your main senaesthetic avenue is, the most conducive method of learning is to concentrate on that experience and move your main focus away from the other senses.

Intuition can be described as the way you interpret the information you have sensed. So, having recognised the subtle information in your environment, you need to understand this in some way. Your intuitive skills will enable you to do this, translating the vibrations around you into usable concepts that you can then communicate to others or use as an insight into the environment around you.

When using your intuition to work in treatments or other areas of interest, you will find that flashes of inspiration or streams of information come to you. Reiki and Ki in general behave in very different ways to our physical world, yet we often interpret things in a very physical way. When we encounter any form of vibrational information, our subconscious mind attempts to translate the information in a way that your conscious mind will understand. Your subconscious works in images and sounds; its linguistic ability is limited to a few words and 'puns'; plus it can only recognise the internal – as far as your subconscious is concerned; only you exist. Every other person in the world is just a part of you!

If you play your subconscious translations through these filters, you will often end up with very different results to the things you started with! So whenever you obtain imagery or other information from your subconscious, I would recommend you always work with that information in the following way:

- Change all 'other people' into aspects of yourself.

- Images either refer to the self, or they will be a play on words.
- 'Inside' (so a car, house, etc.) will mean the body.
- 'Outside' (A landscape, etc.) will refer to energy/Ki.
- Images are often symbolic (Water is emotion, Fire is destruction, Air is life, and so on)
- Subconscious translations will refer to your personal experience.

When we first start to practise with psychic abilities and intuitive thought, we will often receive 'dream-like' information that is mostly image based and symbolic. Yet, as we learn how to translate this more effectively, it will become an automatic process that can be very elaborate and give huge amounts of detailed information.

The Intuitive Ability Exercise

1. Stand in the centre of a room in a quiet place where you will not be disturbed for the duration of the exercise. Centre yourself, close your eyes and bring your focus inwards. Turn your attention completely to your breathing, taking long, slow, deep breaths that cause your stomach to expand and chest to move outwards to the sides. Breathe this way until you start to feel relaxed and very calm – if you feel dizzy or light-headed, sit down for a while until you feel better.

2. Now, place your hands out in front of you, palms facing down and start to project a Celtic Reiki essence, such as Saille or Duir, while pushing downwards through the air. When you reach a resistance, 'sit' your hands on this 'energy cushion' and relax your arms into this resting place. If you wish, you can ask in your

mind for your guides to be with you or ask for assistance from your 'higher-self'. Many people do find additional help very useful at this point and who you ask for this help is entirely up to you. You may want to ask for unseen friends, your loved ones who have passed over, nature spirits or other spiritual beings. You might also decide that you prefer just to work on your own, in which case, ask to connect to your 'higher levels of consciousness'.

3. Now affirm that you will experience 'the vibrations of this location through my subtle senses' and wait for a response. This response should take the form of a slight 'magnetic' pull in your hands, which should direct one or both of your hands to the left/right. You may also find this sensation pulling you forward or backward and do be prepared for this with 'soft knees'. If the pull takes you beyond the comfortable reach of your arms, you can walk slowly in the desired direction. It is important to use the word 'location' rather than saying 'the room' as you are sensing our energetic place as opposed to the physical locale.

4. Search for changes in the vibrations and continue to explore these changes until you find a vibration so 'heavy' that you cannot push through it without using muscle effort. Bounce your hands along these heavy vibrations until you have a good idea of the boundaries. Then push your hands further into the vibrations of energy – if the force is too strong and pushes you back, or resists completely, push the fingertips of your left hand into the barrier, creating a claw with your hand that pierces the energy as opposed to pushing.

5. Once you have done this, ask in your mind,

what 'this' is and then clear your mind as best you can. Allow images, words, feelings, sounds and so on, to fill your mind. You might find it helps at this point to clarify what you perceive by stating aloud your experiences.

6. Upon completing this, come fully back into the room, take a seat and have a moment to compose yourself and make any notes.

The Mastery of Celtic Reiki

A common view of Mastery in any Reiki practice is that of arriving at a stage in your practice where you are mastered by Reiki, which is derived from an equally common notion that the Reiki Master has mastered Reiki. There are some who say it is a Mastery of the practice that counts (which in my perspective is a little akin to saying that somebody is a Master of Electricity because they can work the telly!) So, what exactly is Mastery?

Well, once again, I refer to the philosophy of individual perspective and Mastery being whatever you take it to mean – a title, certification, training to a particular level, so many years of practice, so many clients treated or students trained. However you personally perceive Mastery, those criteria are perfect for you.

My perspective of Mastery is one, literally of perspective – for I believe it is the point of view that creates the Mastery. I have met people who truly deserve the title 'Celtic Reiki Master' even though they have never trained in the system or in some cases, have not even heard of the system! It is due to their utter love of our planet and their deep sense of connection to all living things. Now, I'm not speaking about passion that is disconnected from the Earth – the type of passion that creates hatred for other people because of their actions against our planet; I'm referring to a deep sense of nature at the very core – a realisation that some need to die to support the lives of others, that trees fall and things change. In these people exists a respect for cycles and the knowledge that beyond the physical, a core of complete benevolence reigns.

This understanding extends beyond death, for when we die, our bodies become saturated with endorphins that offer us a sense of total peace, well-being and complete immersion in joy. We see perfection and feel connection in ways that are unlike anything we have ever known. We honestly do save the best for last! This is the same for every living thing, from single-celled organisms to humans and this demonstrates an implicit kindness in the Universe. That whenever and however we die, the experience is an adventure in enlightenment and bliss. Any force – nature, the Universe, Source, God that offers us that comfort, washes away the need for hatred and fear. We do not need to hate those who chop down trees, we just need to love and respect trees ourselves. We need not grieve for the dead, just be kind to the living. There is no need to fear those who kill or harm others, just know that all is as it should be and discover the happiness to be had in each single moment we have.

This is what Celtic Reiki has shown me and I view this attitude as the absolute personification of Mastery. We are not activists, per se, we are custodians. We do not dislike others because of their actions or behaviour, we focus on our own sense of love and deep compassion for all life. We do not see a world of pain and suffering, we know that all is perfect in dynamic and harmony.

With this attitude in place, we instil our perspective into each treatment, Orientation, practice and action we take in our Celtic Reiki practice. We develop our skills, techniques and methodology with a view to constant respect and acceptance that if we want change, we need to look inwards at our own responsibility, rather than outwards towards blame.

I cherish Celtic Reiki, not because of the name or because I was the one who originated the practice. I cherish it because of the wisdom I learnt, the adventures I had, the joy I explored and most of all, for the friends I made. If you want true Mastery of Celtic Reiki, I would recommend looking at these aspects of your practice and yourself – for there you will find your true power and bliss.

The Mastery Begins...

In the following section, we shall investigate a selection of Master treatments, manifestation techniques, teaching tools and advice, as well as some information about essence creation and harvesting. As you dip in and out of these exercises and tutorials, please remember that these tools are not Mastery in the truest sense – they are ways of helping us attain a state of Mastery, just as the hammer and chisel are not the art of Carpentry.

The Master Treatments

These are four Master Treatment methods that were especially created for Celtic Reiki. Based on elemental balance and the alignment of your client, these can be used to provide a greater emphasis on the way the essences of the Woodland Realm work to achieve a specific result. The four treatments are:

- The Breath of Wind
- Raising the Fire
- The Flowing Stream
- Of Earth and Stone

So, let us imagine that your client is so grounded that they have a tendency to create stagnation in their life and cannot move forward; you may choose to use The Flowing Stream to create movement. However, you could also opt for The Breath of Wind to raise the energy-level up and thus offer a feeling of lightness to your client. Also, with these treatments, you might also decide to use Of Earth and Stone to maintain clients grounding while using the uplifting tree essences, such as Saille, Onn or Ailim, for example.

Raising the Fire

This form of treatment is an excellent motivator and invigorator, as it stimulates energy to very high levels thus raising the effectiveness of a treatment with people who tend towards the lowering of vibrations, for example, those who suffer with depression, ME, lethargy, etc. This treatment is particularly expansive for clients who feel great for around two hours after treatment, but then return to the previous state.

A vital aspect to remember with Fire is that, in Eastern philosophy, Fire and Wood are linked as Wood feeds Fire, yet Fire destroys Wood. I have often found this in the treatment as we start with your chosen tree essences that slowly subside to the Tan Essence. Do not worry about the trees, as this does not affect them at all – it is a purely energetic effect of the treatment!

By instilling tree essences at the beginning of the treatment, you will have an effect on your client that is identical to a normal Celtic Reiki treatment using those essences. However, once you raise the fire, the tree elements will give way to a very powerful stimulation of energy (Fire) that will create vigour and dynamic potential in the tree essences. By the completion of the treatment, your client will feel invigorated, yet the tree essences will still be underlying and thus working away to achieve the intent of the treatment.

Therefore, as opposed to a common scenario in these circumstances where the tree essences work for a while before easing back to the previous state, here the fire will keep your client's energy levels high so that the tree essences can work for longer and more efficiently.

The routine:

1. Start with your usual opening routine, centring yourself, asking your helpers (if you have them) and creating a connection with your client.

2. Now, state internally, this is to be a "Raising the Fire Treatment".

3. Stand at your client's head, with your hands at their temples and activate your chosen Woodland Realm essences either as a Treatment Forest or in a Woodhenge.

4. Once you have a good sense of the essences, just relax and let the energy build. Remain for 10 minutes at the head area and then for a further 10 minutes on the shoulders.

5. Now move to the side of your client and complete a further 10 minutes with one hand over your subject's heart and the other at the base (pelvic) area.

6. 30 minutes into the treatment, you begin to Raise the Fire with the activation of Tan.

7. Imagine your hands are resting on a carpet of energy, just above your client, in a position, so you are resting your arms comfortably on this carpet as opposed to holding them there. Relax your shoulders.

8. Now allow your arms and hands to move along

the perceived waves of magnetism, going to whatever area of your subject's body or aura they wish to move to. Whilst doing this, imagine flames of energy glowing with the colours of the rainbow, flickering up from your client's body to meet your hands. Feel the heat of these flames against the palms of your hands.

9. Continue this for a further 20-30 minutes, seeing the flames becoming more and more vibrant as they completely encompass your subject and glow brighter and brighter.

10. At the end of the treatment, make a final 'head connection' with your client (hands on the temples), thank those who helped you and then work through any usual closing routine that you have.

11. Bring your subject into the room, make sure they are lucid and then offer them some water to drink!

The Breath of Wind

This technique uses the element of Air to create an energy dynamic that is gentle, yet multifaceted in effect, and all-encompassing. The routine is very relaxing, for both the client and the practitioner, as you gently stimulate your client's energetic systems with Celtic Reiki essences, your breath, and slow, repetitive movements. Particularly good for people with lots of stress and tension, the Breath of Wind helps people to lift upwards and focus forwards, as opposed as focussing themselves into the ground.

This is an excellent method for people who are 'too grounded' and look only to the physical for every solution and when making decisions. I have also found this form of treatment works well on the symptoms of dis-eases create as a result of this attitude. These can be, but are not limited to, cancer, neurological illness, hypertension and the effects caused by heart-attack or stroke. The technique is also wonderful for people who are 'stuck' emotionally, or in states where they lack emotion or experience emotional stagnation – such as people stuck in relationships or life situations that are no longer serving them in beneficial ways.

The Wind rustles the branches and leaves of the trees, enabling them to sing to each other and communicate using murmured messages that are carried on the breeze. Hence, this method can also be valuable when wanting to stimulate the creativity of energy, causing it to 'sing' with vibrancy or to work with affirmations for your subject that can be formed through the initial consultation, or through the use of affirmation cards.

The Routine:

1. Start with your favoured opening routine, centring yourself and asking your helpers (if you have them) and making a connection with your client.

2. In your mind, state that this is to be a "Breath of Wind Treatment".

3. Stand at your subject's head, with your hands at their temples and activate your chosen essences as a Treatment Forest or in the Woodhenge.

4. Once you have a good sense of energy, just relax and let the energy build, holding conscious attention on the rhythm of your breathing. Take long slow breaths, whilst visualising yourself pulling in the energy of Annal and exhaling this energy on your breath. This should be blown out through your mouth so slowly and gently that your subject cannot feel it, yet it acts like the wind in their energy field.

5. Continue this for 10 minutes, easing your breath if you become faint or dizzy. Then continue at the shoulders for a further 10 minutes.

6. Now, remaining at your subject's head area, lift your hands so that they are about 12 inches above their head, palms facing downwards. Then slowly sweep the air down the length of their body so that your arms stretch forward completely and your palms are facing away from you – breathe out as you do this. Breathe in and return your palms to their original position. Repeat for 10 minutes.

7. Then go to the side of your subject and stand at the midpoint of their body, around the lower abdomen. Place your hands, palms down, at

their head area and then breathing out as you do so, sweep your hands slowly, steadily and gently down the length of your subject's body until you reach their feet (or as close as you can get to their feet without moving). Breathe in as you return your hands to the head area and pull in Annal as you do so.

8. After 10 minutes, go down to your client's feet and repeat the exercise listed in (6) the head area section, except this time, come up the body with your sweeping hands. Do this for 10 minutes.

9. Now go to the other side of your client and stand at their midpoint. Place your hands palms facing down at your subject's feet (or as best you can without overreaching) and slowly sweep energy up their body to their head (or as near as you can). Breathe out as you do this and breathe in as you return your hands to the feet.

10. At the end of the treatment, make a final head connection with your subject (hands on the temples), silently express your gratitude and then work through your usual closing routine.

11. Bring your subject into the room, make sure they are lucid, and then offer them some water.

The Flowing Stream

The stream constantly flows in a natural movement downhill, creating energy dynamics that are vibrant, yet focussed in one direction. The Flowing Stream is thus an excellent choice for those who require Celtic Reiki treatments with a directional intent – so you can use the essences as a way to focus on a particular issue or area.

Examples of this could be using Coll, Phagos and Nuin in a Stream Treatment for somebody who is facing impeding exams or maybe Luis, Tinne, Duir and Onn for those who require the ability to assert themselves against one particular person or situation (a violent partner or aggressive boss for instance).

The Flowing Stream also guides those who have lost their direction in life and fallen by the wayside on their path. It helps gather momentum, but in a specific way as opposed to the random direction and dynamics of Air. The Water always flows towards the sea. In this respect the Sea becomes the goal, the stream is the path and the Celtic Reiki essences are the boat in which you travel.

Excellent for use in manifestation treatments, particularly where the manifestation is a state of mind, health or emotional state: examples of these could be 'Inner Peace', 'Joy', 'Abundance', 'Healthy', 'Rested', 'Enlightened', etc. You can also use The Flowing Stream for the fluid systems of the body such as the circulatory or lymphatic systems.

The Routine:

1. Begin with your preferred opening, centring yourself, asking for help and guidance if you wish it and making a connection with your client.
2. Internally state that this is to be a "Flowing Stream Treatment".
3. Stand at your subject's head with your hands

at their temples and activate your chosen tree prescription either as a Treatment Forest or in the Woodhenge.

4. Once you have a definite feeling of energy, just relax and let the energy build, experiencing the essences of Celtic Reiki throughout your body. Start to become the energy, allowing the potency of Dwr to well up through the base of your spine, through your lower abdomen, shoulders, the cascades down through your arms. Remember to keep 'soft knees' during this entire treatment.

5. When you are ready, start to move around your subject, as and when you intuit, all the time maintaining this level of energy – you are the stream, flowing through your subject, washing away their pain, focusing their energy, enabling them to flow with you.

6. Complete this treatment, going with the flow for an hour, or as long as you think is necessary to attain the intent of the session.

7. At the end of the treatment, create the final head connection with your client by placing your hands, lightly on their temples. Thank those who have assisted you and then work through any usual closing routine that you have.

8. Bring your subject into the room, make sure they are lucid, and then offer them some water to drink.

Of Earth and Stone

This magical, Father Earth based technique is grounding, yet it does not necessarily work by grounding the subject – I have found it is more likely to ground the Celtic Reiki treatment with the client, thus having a more integral affect. So this could suggest that when treating somebody who is overly grounded, you could work with a 'head' orientated tree, such as Saille or Gort and use Of Earth and Stone to ground those essences within your client. This would not ground them any further, but would instead lift them to a deeply grounded but 'lighter' energy.

As with The Flowing Stream, this technique is excellent for manifestation purposes, except here the focus is on material or physical manifestation, such as finances, property, a home, a soul mate, more time, etc. I have also perceived this treatment as very beneficial to the supportive structures of the body such as the skeletal and muscular systems as well as all the internal organs.

With use of the Standing Stones and their connection to the earth and past, this method can be used not only for physically-centred treatments and magic, but for yielding wonderful results in connecting to the past, both karmic and ancestral. Thus you can deal with past life issues and with disease or trauma that has been suffered by a person's relatives and by humanity in the wider sense. So, if you know your client's grandmother died of heart failure, you could use Gort (heart), Ioho (Death) and Of Earth and Stone to clear the dynamic that caused this death – I believe this means that there is less chance of your client succumbing to this vibrational 'miasm'. You could do this on the wider picture too, for example using Luis (Immune System), Tinne (Sexual Disease), Coll (Boosts Physical/Emotional Healing) and Sycamore (Acceptance) to help ease the world of the HIV/AIDS pandemic

The Routine:

1. Initiate the treatment with your favoured opening routine, centring yourself, asking for guidance if you have unseen helpers or of the trees and make a connection with your client.

2. Now state with your inner voice that this is to be an "Of Earth and Stone Treatment".

3. Stand at the head area of your client, with your hands at their temples and activate your chosen essences of the Woodland or Standing Stones Realms either as a Woodhenge or a Stonehenge.

4. When you can feel the Celtic Reiki essences, just relax and let the energy build and take your attention to your subject's feet at the opposite end of the treatment couch. Visualise a pillar of Pridd essence rising up to the same height as you are, just below your subject's feet. Then see two more pillars rise up, one at either side of your subject (at '3 o'clock' and '9 o'clock').

5. Then visualise eight more pillars of Pridd, in between the existing pillars and you, so that you have a circle of standing stones that look like the face of a clock if you were to be looking down from the ceiling. Now feel the Pridd energy rise up through your feet, completing the circle, as you become the 12th standing stone.

6. Now spend between 3-5 minutes at each point in the standing stone circle and as you stand at the location of each stone, place your hands on, or above your client – you may find the circle is elongated, like an oval, but this does not matter.

7. At the end of the treatment, make a final head connection by placing your hands gentle on or either side of your client's temples, thank those

who helped you and then work through any usual closing routine that you have.

8. As with all treatments, ask your client to come back into the room, make sure they are lucid, and then offer them some water to drink.

The Manifestation Techniques

The Grove of Creation

With this technique, you can conduct the processes and visualisations both for self-treatment, or when treating others. The only difference being that your client may possibly be in the room with you when you conduct the latter.

It is purely an individual choice, but you may like to involve your client consciously, by walking them through the visualisations.

One thing you may notice in the method laid out below is the lack of prescription (which essences to use), this is because the true meaning of manifestation is to state what you want and then heal the different aspects of yourself that are stopping you from obtaining that goal. There really is no difference between healing and manifestation! Therefore, the essences you use are down to what you intuit you should use and how you think they should be placed as opposed to using 'this tree' for 'that purpose'.

To help you with this, we work with two tree guides: The Lord of Thorns and Sanctuary Oak. They will offer a sacred space to conduct the manifestation treatment and help you intuit which essences to use and when.

The Routine:

1. Prepare yourself for the treatment by centring yourself, closing your eyes, focusing on your breathing and then completing any opening routines that you personally enjoy.
2. Now ask the Lord of Thorns and Sanctuary Oak to be with you.
3. Standing at your client's head area, stand with your back straight, feet firmly on the floor and knees slightly bent. Make a head connection by placing your hands on or over your client's temples and await a good sense of connection between you.
4. Now state the intent of the manifestation treatment, i.e., what it is that you or your client wishes to manifest. Then trigger the essence(s) you feel necessary; in the original version of Celtic Reiki, this would primarily be Nuin.
5. Now visualise a sacred grove in front of you, seeing two large trees creating a gateway – let the images flow and do not try to force them. If you find it easier to create a sense of imagery by hearing or feeling, listen to the sound of the wind in the leaves or explore the trunks of the trees with your internal senses, imagining what they would feel like to the touch. It is important to remember, energetically you are actually in the grove and that it is not imagined!
6. Now, with this scene firmly in your mind, place your hands on your lap for self treatment or on your client's shoulders. Then, in your mind's

eye, see yourself leading them through the 'gateway trees' and into a sacred sanctuary, deep in the heart of the grove.

7. In this sacred space are a group of trees that form a circle all around you – there can be as many or a little as you like, although 12 is a good number as you can base the layout on the face of a clock. Each tree should be relevant to your purpose and you can have many trees of one species if you wish. You may find that you do not recognise what some of the trees are, or you may want to use a tree that you have not physically encountered before, so cannot visualise it accurately – neither of these considerations matter, as the exercise will work regardless.

8. In the centre of the circle, see the Lord of Thorns – a regal holly tree, and The Sanctuary Oak – a strong and powerful Oak tree with his limbs outstretched to nurture. Keep your assertion of energy strong and guide your client towards the Holy and Oak, stating the intent for this treatment.

9. Now all the trees begin to glow with light, getting brighter and brighter as the treatment is conducted, the light gets so bright in fact, that you feel waves of energy begin projected towards you from every tree. Breathe in this energy and project it through your client using your out-breath to help focus the Celtic Reiki and your manifestation intent.

10. Now you may either stay at the client's head/shoulder area, or move around them, depending on what your preference is. All the time, try to maintain the image of the grove in your mind, until your subject starts to glow with the energy too.

11. At the end of the treatment (which can last between thirty minutes and an hour depending on what time you have set aside), thank the trees in turn and any higher guidance that you have previously asked to help you. Then lead your subject back through the gateway and then close down in whatever way you intuit.

12. Ask your client to return to the room, check that they are fully-awake, and offer them a glass of water.

You can also adapt this treatment to work as a self-treatment by imagining yourself on the treatment couch and conducting the routine with the proviso that you receive the treatment when you lay on the couch – then lay down on the couch for an hour to reconnect with the energy. I like to view this technique as reflecting two parts of the self – the Master Aspect who conducts the treatment and the Client Aspect who receives it.

You can also conduct a self-treatment by simply sitting in a chair and running through the meditation for yourself, by yourself

The Ocean of Possibilities

This treatment uses various elements of the Mor Essence plus others to create a dual layer treatment that is visualised by both subject and practitioner, along with energy work that is connected to the treatment space in support of the visualisation. You may wish to record your visualised inner journey before using this technique so that you can simply playback the steps during the treatment and both you and your client can follow the instructions on your recording.

The treatment will last about 20-30 minutes when just using the visualisation as a time guide, so if you do want to conduct a longer treatment, simply add an additional 20-40 minutes of Celtic Reiki essence connection after the visualisation to produce a greater integrity of bond to the goal and intent. Try to intuit the tree essences that will be of most use to the individual goals and desires of the manifestation.

The Routine:

1. Prepare yourself for the treatment, by centring yourself, closing your eyes, and focusing on your breathing. Then use any opening rituals that you personally enjoy.

2. Now ask for your unseen friends to be with you, or conduct the introductory connections you usually carry out at the beginning of a treatment.

3. Moving to your client's head area, stand with your back straight, feet firmly on the floor, and with knees slightly bent. Create a connection to your client by placing your hands on or over their temple area awaiting a strong sense of energy between you.

4. Now state the intent of the manifestation treatment, i.e., what it is that your client wants to manifest. Then activate Mor – with a

visualisation of the essence connecting to you, your client and then filling the room completely.

5.   Having felt the intense vibrancy of the Mor essence all around you, connect to Bearn (Space) and visualise this above you for a couple of minutes.

6.   Look to your client's feet and stimulate Pridd (Earth) just below their feet to ground their desires to the Earth.

7.   Then look to your client's left and stimulate Tan (Fire) to their left hand side, in order to activate their spiritual and creative energy.

8.   Now turn to your subject's right hand side and here trigger Annal (Air) to help them free their logical and practical mind from limiting belief.

9.   Where you stand at their head, connect to the Dwr (Water) essence, imagine these as drops of rain that carry the dreams and intents of your client to manifestation and fruition.

10. Now holding all of these images in your mind for a moment, then begin the inner journey and visualise this as you are talking your client through the process.

11. Visualise the ocean and your subject gently floating on the ocean's surface – they are perfectly safe and just rest, bobbing around. Then start to send down an energetic link to the very bottom of the sea – travel deeper; further and further into the dark, connecting to the ocean floor and then going into the earth itself, enabling the energy of the earth to immerse your client.

12. Now return to your subject on the surface and feel the gentle breeze from their right blowing against their body and the heat from the sun on their left hand side, try to instil a real feeling of this in your client. Then ask them to see the blue sky above, free of clouds.

13. Now ask your subject to visualise the focus of their manifestation goal and ask them to do this, to see various objects rise to the surface of the water and bob about – these could be anything from bits of wood, to household objects, plants, statues, even whole buildings, or islands. Let whatever needs to come to the surface, come – these are the things that are blocking your subject from getting what they want.

14. After several minutes, ask your client to feel the direction they need to move in, then get them to move away and release all of these items. Get them to swim gently away from these blockages and find a place where they are free from the things that stop them, or hold them back.

15. Now a golden cloud gently comes into view and little droplets of golden rain start to fall upon their face, bringing their dreams to them, manifesting their goals and enabling them to get what they want.

16. Get them to sense the rain with all five senses (see it, hear it, taste, it, smell it, and feel it) and gradually ask them to see the entire ocean turning gold as their dreams start to become reality.

17. Once this is done, either bring your client back into the room, or continue with a tree essence treatment.

18. Finally, check that your client is fully awake, and offer them a glass of water, before asking them to sit back in a chair.

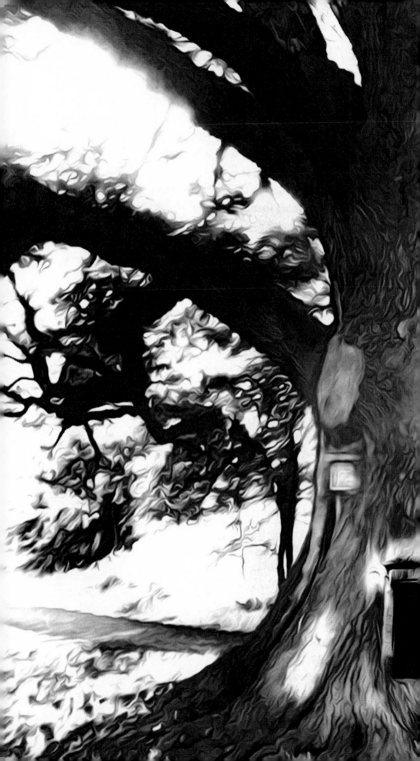

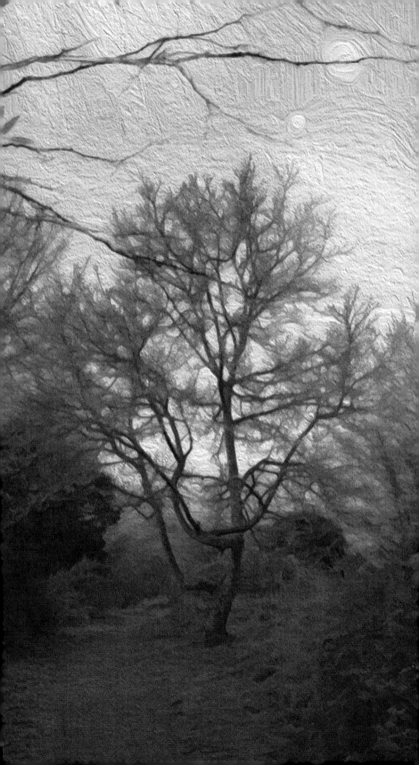

The Path to Teaching Celtic Reiki

Teaching Celtic Reiki can be one of the most rewarding and humbling experiences you can encounter. The indescribable pleasure of seeing your students undergoing such profound transformation and attaining bliss in their connection to Reiki, to the trees, and the Earth is completely awe-inspiring.

The ability to share your experiences, your perspective and your own, close connection to the Earth is the rather plump cherry on top of a multifaceted, multilayered cake. Yet the wonder does not cease here—for there are the unexpected effects of teaching: the amazing experience of Orientation; witnessing your students Calibration and feeling it with them, every step of the way; the reaction of the trees to you as you teach others and how the world becomes different; and the sheer bliss of creating friendship, based on shared passion and innate love of life.

Since 2013, only currently licensed Realm Masters are accredited to teach others, meaning that previously qualified Celtic Reiki Masters need to update their qualification. This assures the quality and professionalism of teaching in our therapy.

Therefore, what follows is a mere sliver of the tools we use to achieve the basis of our teaching methods. What I am unable to write here is the indefinable transcendence of words and concepts this spectrum of techniques can proffer when use together as part of your training delivery and Master Teacher adventure...

The Ki Classroom: A Grove Sanctuary

A major difference between traditional Reiki practices and Celtic Reiki is that the newer styles of Celtic Reiki replicate the nature of Ki, as opposed to following a method of linear components that I feel are very 'un-energetic' in nature. In Usui Reiki we viewed a class as part theory, part attunement, part practical, with elements such as 'clearing the room of negative energy', and teaching our students inadvertently, how to divorce themselves from an energetic view by using terms such as 'channel', 'protect', 'taking on energy', and so on.

In Celtic Reiki we attempt to interact with our students in the same way that Reiki interacts with us – in a completely integrated way where one is not separated from the other. To do this, we create the 'Ki classroom', in which we are immersed within a specific environment and in this place teaching and learning become completely indiscernible from each other.

The Ki Classroom is essentially a consciously defined integration of the various learning layers that occur in a Celtic Reiki practice workshop. This means that Orientation and Calibration are continuous throughout the day(s), or sessions and run in fluidity with the academic and practical training. With your Koad facet in place at the very beginning of the class, there is no need for cleansing, or preparation of the Ki 'in the room', because you are basically not working within the physical environment.

Once you have set up your Koad (Grove), you then begin the class with a brief introductory session and an overview of the course syllabi. Then it is time to create the symbiotic relationship with your students, which is described in the following section of this chapter. From this point onwards, you are merely an onlooker in the Celtic Reiki teaching processes, as the energetic realms just beyond your perception start to interact with those outside of your students' awareness and you all begin to expand your awareness to those areas.

In this energetic sanctuary, you, the teacher, become a symbiotic being that is multifaceted, multidimensional, and intangible. No longer do we deem ourselves to be a single person who is teaching a class, instead we choose to become the interaction of our students between themselves and each other. Each word we say in our Ki classroom is not a single word, but a word multiplied by the number of students that we have in the classroom. You are the meeting of your students with themselves and when you speak, it is your students teaching themselves their truth, their wisdom.

'You' no longer exist outside the physical form, enabling your various facets to become the classroom and absorb the information that is contained within. Hence, as your students teach themselves Celtic Reiki, you learn how to perceive Reiki through their eyes and their perspectives. Thus, the Celtic Reiki methodology becomes clearer to you, sharper, more comprehensible. When you return to being 'you' at the end of the workshop, you will have expanded your sphere of perception beyond what it was before, not in a linear way, but in a multidimensional sense.

Using this approach, the various subliminal Calibrations that take place when you activate Koad, filter through into physicality during the course of the session and form a seamless integration of Ki with the Orientations that you conduct during the workshop.

Your Ki Classroom thus offers a totally unique, yet completely immersive experience for your students, less comparable with the traditional way of teaching and more in line with our current energetic experience.

Example Syllabus Using a Ki Classroom...

- Workshop and group introduction
- Explain the syllabus
- Creation of the Ki Classroom Meditation
- Administration
- Initial theory and questions
- Orientation and Calibration
- Break
- Theory
- Lunch
- Additional Ki Classroom Meditation
- Orientation and Calibration
- Introduction to Practical Techniques
- Practical Techniques
- Break
- Practical Techniques
- Questions
- Conclusion and End

Creating Your Ki Classroom

The creation of the Ki Classroom starts prior to the arrival of your students and consists of the following process:

1. Stand in the centre of the room and look at the corners of the room, both at floor and ceiling height. Connect to the physicality of these corners and then centre yourself, close your eyes and stand comfortably, with your feet firmly on the floor, soft knees, and shoulder relaxed.

2. Take a few deep, slow breaths into your lower abdomen and then activate the Koad facet of Reiki by saying "Koad, Koad, Koad" and visualising the Ogham symbol if required.

3. Feel yourself adjusting to the Grove, lifting the physicality of the room into a Grove Ki State as you do so.

4. Come back into the room.

The next step is conducted in the initial section of your class and takes the form of a meditation that you walk your students through.

1. Sit facing your students and ask them to sit comfortably, with their feet firmly on the floor, eyes closed, and shoulders relaxed.

2. Ask the apprentices to take several deep breaths, into their lower abdomen and expanding to the sides. As you do this, turn your attention to each student and focus upon him or her for a moment.

3. Activate the Koad Facet of Reiki.

4. Ask your students to clear their minds and focus only on their breathing, whilst you take your attention to the left hemisphere of your brain. Look up to the left for a moment and then

pull your attention back into your head, until you reach the occipital region. Then move into the centre of your head and wait for a moment.

5. Ask your students to focus on the left hemisphere just as you have done. Then get them to take some more deep breaths.

6. Take your attention to the right hemisphere of your brain. Look up to the right for a moment and then pull your attention back into your head, until you reach the occipital region.

7. Ask your students to focus on the right hemisphere just as you have done. Then get them to take some more deep breaths.

8. Now close your eyes, look up and to the left, then up and to the right, return your eyes to centre and move backwards through the centre of your head. Activate the Unhewn Dolman Arch Facet of Reiki (UDA) and feel Reiki expanding outwards from this point.

9. Ask your students to look to the left, right, centre and then move backwards through the head. You may see them pull backwards at this point; this is a good sign of connection, so ask them not to resist any pulling.

10. Expand your UDA Reiki through your body then look at each student in turn, feel the shift of energy as you do this.

11. Bring your students back into the room.

There is no need to disconnect from the Ki Classroom, however it is advisable to conduct a shortened version of the above routine when you return from the lunch break (if applicable). This abbreviated technique consists of steps 1, 2, 3, 8, 9, 10, and 11.

1. Sit facing your students and ask them to sit comfortably, with their feet firmly on the floor, eyes closed, and shoulders relaxed.

2. Asked them to take several deep breaths, into their lower abdomen and expanding to the sides. As you do this, turn your attention to each student and focus upon him or her for a moment.

3. Activate the Koad Facet of Reiki.

4. Now close your eyes, look up and to the left, then up and to the right, return your eyes to centre and move backwards through the centre of your head. Activate the UDA Essence and feel Reiki expanding outwards from this point.

5. Ask your students to look to the left, right, centre and then move backwards through the head. You may see them pull backwards at this point; this is a good sign of connection, so ask them not to resist any pulling.

6. Expand the UDA through your body then look at each student in turn, feel the shift of energy as you do this.

7. Bring your students back into the room.

The Woodland Path

The Woodland Path is a Master Teacher tool that spans the entire duration of a workshop or course. This could be over the two day period of an event, or over several months for those studying remotely.

Each Woodland Path consists of a band of specific essences that work on the basis of a cycle (this is the 'Path'). During the completion of a single cycle there may be various points at which the cycle stops and some type of healing takes place. This could be the healing of some form of disease, a limiting belief, or some other barrier to the student's progress. Whether this synthesis is to heal a trauma, or to boost the energy of a specific aspect of the student's experience, these stopping points trigger the application of the essences or 'Trees' that form the 'Woodland'. At the beginning of a student's training or the start of a course, you connect each of your Apprentices to their Woodland Paths, so their energy systems (along with other cerebral and physiological systems) travel the path, growing, healing and evolving with each Tree that is passed.

Once the cycle is completed, it begins again, but this time from a different perspective, so what appears to be a continuous circle of vibrations, is actually a spiral that will expand their knowledge and skills for the entire duration of their training, making knowledge retention easier, confidence greater and energy work more effective. On your Celtic Reiki training, you will be shown how to use Woodland Paths, although a simplified version is included here for your interest.

Creating Your Woodland Paths

You may wish to complete this technique as part of the Ki Classroom process, or you could conduct the Woodland Path creation by itself or as part of a guided meditation. If you are a Master of some other form of Reiki modality and wish to incorporate the Woodland Path into your classes, you can adapt this technique by using the Master Essences of your particular style in place of the Celtic Reiki Essences listed here. If you are not a Reiki Master, but have had some training or you are just curious, try creating a Woodland Path for yourself using essences or intent. You could, for example, create a Path to help you achieve some goal or task.

1. Take a few moments to centre yourself in the room, or environment.
2. Take several deep breaths, focussing on your diaphragm, ensuring that you expand your lower abdomen to the sides with each in breath.
3. Hold your hands out in front of you, shoulders relaxed and your hands held straight out, fingers pointing away from your body and palms facing each other (as if you are holding an invisible box in front of your body).
4. Hold the image of the cube in your hands and slowly send it into your lower abdomen.
5. Trigger "Woodland Path" as per your usual triggering style.
6. Send a circle of Woodland Path Essence from the cube and encircle your Apprentice completely, before returning the Path to the cube. This creates a complete cycle, extending from and to the cube, where your student(s) exist within the circle and you stand at the point of origination.
7. Trigger 'Koad'.
8. Raise the Woodland Path to match this essence.
9. Come back into the room completely and then bring your students into the room.

Teaching with Orientation and Calibration

When preparing your students for the Calibration to an Orientation, it is advisable to ensure that you have comfortable seats for them to sit on, but not so relaxing that they are enticed into sleep. Also ensure that seating is of a height suitable for you to place your hands around people's heads/on shoulders, without bending over or stretching too far. Also ensure that you have cushions for people's feet should they not be able to reach the floor. As you are about to start the process, check that everybody has his or her spine straight, and head up – try to stop any slouching, etc.

Remember to explain, prior to the Orientation, the types of sensation people are likely to experience. Remember to keep your language very positive and upbeat at all times, focussing on the synaesthesia responses that commonly occur during the Calibration.

After the Orientation, change the pace, pitch, and volume of your voice, which should have been soft, quiet, and slow at the beginning of the process, becoming quick, loud, and deep as you get students back into the room.

CONSIDERATIONS FOR THE MASTERTEACHER

When starting to teach Celtic Reiki, the workshop preparation begins long before the class ever comes to fruition and there are distinctions that should be made from the outset: There are three areas for consideration and preparation: the first is preparation for teaching and ensuring your skills for taking the class are honed and ready; next is the preparation for a course, or workshop in the form of venue, promotion, booking, and so on; and finally the preparation of the individual class in the creation of a framework and syllabus.

The first factor is something to be worked towards at the very beginning of your path as a Celtic Reiki teacher and once you are teaching classes, only need be re-evaluated from time to time, to ensure that your training needs are met and your methods up to date. Preparing to be a teacher is something of a misnomer, as nothing really prepares you for the nervousness and exhilaration of your first class, however being as sure as you can be that you have done the best you can will create a 'step-up'.

The very first thing to do, is to read through your Celtic Reiki course materials while making notes and testing yourself on what the techniques are and how they work. As you work through each step of the course, try to remove yourself from the role of student, being guided by the notes and attempt to make the words your own. How would you express each section of the training as somebody who has used these techniques for themselves and with others? Monitor the places where you have taken what is written for granted and question everything. Try to ask the questions your students may ask and give answers.

Reading your notes as a student is a very different practice to working with them as a teacher, as you are looking to understand the contents from viewpoints other than your own and this time around, you are the guide! As a student it is very easy to repeat things verbatim, without questioning and just trusting the processes. As a teacher, you should understand the inner-workings and unseen elements of the course, the manuals, and the dynamics of Celtic Reiki.

The focus of this exercise is not to refresh your memory – it is to make Celtic Reiki your own: to take what has been written in one person's perspective and to discover your individual view of the techniques. For just as each practitioner has a unique view on his or her Celtic Reiki practice, so does each teacher. The clients who are drawn to you, come, because they are suited to you as a therapist, rather than the therapy you offer, which is just a 'hook'. As a teacher, the student may want to learn Celtic Reiki, but you are their inspiration! You can only be an inspiration when you are speaking your own truth, as opposed to speaking another's ideals word for word.

I make my own course materials available for Celtic Reiki Masters through the nrg organisation (nrgology.com) and these can be printed and used without the need for any writing on your part. These notes provide a good grounding in the history, philosophies, etc. of Celtic Reiki and save a lot of the background work and duplication for any Master.

However, I do suggest that each Master write their own notes – either as a main course manual or as an accompanying booklet for the nrg notes. These will be very personal to each teacher and offer your own perspective of Essences, techniques and styles that you favour, along with your views on Celtic philosophy, Reiki and so on.

A valuable way of working with Celtic Reiki from the perspective of a teacher is to basically deconstruct the course and then rebuild it, either as a complete course, or as 'small chunks'. So you may decide that rather than constructing a two-day practitioner workshop, you create a ten week course that focuses on the practical treatment techniques and consultation methods. You may also decide to add elements from other therapies that you are qualified to work with, such as massage, or life coaching.

The deconstruction of a subject for the purposes of teaching it to others can be lengthy, but is very worthwhile. As you pull something apart and then remake it in your own way, you create a process. It is this process that is valuable, as it can be transferred to others more easily than something that you have learnt on a face-value basis.

Another beneficial result in deconstruction is that you can ask yourself at each step, how you can shift the focus of the course to those people that you wish to teach. So a child will require a very different type of Celtic Reiki course from a teenager, adult, and so on. As you isolate each section of the course, ask yourself who you are aiming your courses and workshops at, and how they are likely to respond to the technique/area you are covering. Try not to categorise too much, but see this as a method of gaining an insight, as opposed to hard and fast rules.

You can also use this time to write some notes of your own, either as additions to the provided Celtic Reiki manuals or as the basis for your own Celtic Reiki notes in the future. There is so much to achieve when starting out as a teacher of Celtic Reiki that it can often be a real benefit to have the pre-written notes to offer students, although many teachers do wish to write their own notes eventually. There is no obligation to use nrg notes, or indeed, to write your own, the purpose of the pre-written notes is a teacher-support that can free up your time to work on getting your classes up and running with the minimum amount of commotion!

The next process is to practise the teaching experience as a role play, in which you set up a class room environment with everything you need, including chairs, clipboards, notepads, pens, tables, and so on. Then work through each module, practising how you would teach the relevant techniques and theories. You can work from the manuals or your notes on them and remember to make notes of things that you encounter along the way. You may 'hear' questions as you explain something, or have a thought about some other area you want to check. Sometimes, when things are flowing, you may have a flash of inspiration, or eloquence – be sure to write these down too!

Working with the role-playing exercises is particularly useful when it comes to working with any areas of the workshops that you did not resonate with. If there were indeed, sections of Celtic Reiki practice that you feel did not 'sit' as well as you had hoped, it is very likely, you will gain a deeper insight into these techniques through the reflective eyes of others. So, practise with your imaginary class, and see if this distils the elements further for when you come to teaching in a live environment.

The format and type of class that you teach in the future will also depend on personal factors, such as other work commitments, family, and personal circumstances; as you will often need to fit classes around your other responsibilities.

Your Courses and Workshops

The initial factors when deciding on your class format are the times when you can commit to teaching and availability on the larger scale. So, are you able to commit to weekly slots on a certain day throughout the year, or are individual dates a better option for you? If you have good availability throughout the year, you may wish to run several courses, while reasons such as children's school holidays may require you to stop holding courses at certain times.

When you have determined the format of the class you can then create the themes and elements of the course, thus choosing what will be covered on your 'bespoke' classes. The Celtic Reiki course materials come already formatted and so do not require this step. Simply list the elements of the course you feel appropriate and then add any notes to techniques and activities that you can include in the course.

When you add elements to your proposed workshop, or course, you may discover that some techniques work better with regularity and a defined routine of daily/weekly practice. When this happens it could be that you redefine what is covered in the course, shift the perspective of the course, or change the format. It may therefore be feasible to offer your students the 'tools they need to create change' over the one day, rather than 'guiding them through the processes of creating change' which may require a weekly course, and so on.

When creating your classes, you will also have other considerations, such as the available space for students. This will establish the boundaries of how many people can attend the course and have knock-on effects as to the cost-effectiveness of a venue, etc. A good rule of thumb is that Celtic Reiki workshops be kept to small groups of 4-8 people.

Very often, local education centres are looking for Reiki practice teachers to provide and teach their own classes. This can be challenging, as group sizes tend to be large and course durations are usually, but not necessarily, many weeks (12+). The real advantage with teaching these evening classes is that you can offer become involved in Adult Education Teacher Training Programmes and because a qualified teacher.

So with your venue in mind, you can decide on group sizes, workshop contents, and the kind of people your courses are aimed towards. With these considerations taken care of, you can book a date and create promotional material. It is a good idea in the beginning, to arrange a venue that is cheap in price and have a long booking period.

During this period, you can concentrate on writing the notes for your bespoke workshops and courses. At first I would advise that you run a more standard format of course as, in the initial stages of becoming a teacher, this will help free up time for role-playing and offer a tried and trusted framework.

Attempting to write a course, having never taught is very challenging!! Nevertheless, if you wish to write and present your own workshops, a good few months between arranging the course and taking it, will present you with enough time to work on your notes and a deadline to assist your motivation.

Creating Your Course Notes & Timetable

When it comes to writing notes, you will discover your own style and format with practice. Over time you will edit, revise and rewrite your notes to evolve with your teaching style and personal experience. Initially when writing your notes, however, you can focus on a narrative style, or the more straightforward 're-cap style', in which you simply revisit the techniques and tools.

The choice is yours. Remember to keep in mind the oral traditions of Celtic Reiki and where possible, favour the journal or personal experience over the prescriptive methodology. I personally do use step-by-step frameworks, yet these are always presented as learning tools, as opposed to definitive methods or 'rules'.

The costs of printing and binding notes should also be incorporated into your costing estimates when deciding what to charge students for the course and will differ greatly between privately run courses and those taught in Adult Education Facilities.

When writing your notes/manuals, the deconstruction and role-playing exercises will form a valuable basis for your focus and this should be in conjunction with the next area of consideration: the syllabi and structures of your classes.

Structuring your Classes

From your initial overview of the elements and techniques that you want to include in your class, you can now develop a structure that is greater in detail and forms the foundation of your syllabus. This process is usually completed in conjunction with the note writing, as the notes are a place where you can cover the main themes of the class, list suggestions for completing techniques, and add any additional information that you do not intend to include in the class itself.

When you come to structuring your class, it is very much a case of estimation and role-playing with a clock nearby to see that you have time enough to incorporate all the topics you wish to cover. Start with your initial framework and then allocate a running order, trying to find a good flow, so that each element flows into the next. Integrate your exercises, so that you minimise large chunks of either talking, or student exercises. In this way, you will ensure there is a good balance of interaction.

Start with an introduction and group interaction at the beginning of each workshop – this can be in the form of the group familiarising themselves with each other on their first meeting, or reconciliation of work done between workshops if on a longer-term course. Where possible, try to encourage discussion about topics covered and work done, always ensuring that this is done in a supportive and positive way. Set approximate time limits for exercises and ensure that during these times, you sit back and watch, whilst not being intrusive.

I, personally, prefer to set three levels of timetable: minimum, preferred and additional. The minimum timetable runs under time, however this is very useful if you have a group that asks lots of questions and prefers discussion over listening. The preferred timetable is my ideal and comes in on time and finally the additional timetable consists of the preferred elements, plus some extras for when you find yourself with extra time – I have never had to use this timetable, yet still keep it just in case!

It is often a good idea with Celtic Reiki workshops to conduct a meditation before starting any teaching, as this gives you the chance to connect to the facets of your students and shift yourself into the appropriate state. You can also use this time to activate and connect your students to the Ki Classroom.

Conclude the workshops with summary, discussion, questions/answers, feedback, and conclusions, which often take the form of looking forward to the future, either by way of future study, or homework for the week. It is often a good idea to provide feedback forms for your students to complete, so that you can adapt and hone the courses you run, based on helpful feedback.

Once you have created the framework, jot down a syllabus, with rough timings and run this through a role-play, ensuring that you run to schedule and thus, get a feel of the overall class. Of course, you do not need to actually role-play your students exercise times, hence moving directly from one section of your tutoring, to the next.

The dynamics of the classroom environment are such that you can rarely prepare for every eventuality. However, the foundation of a clearly defined framework, syllabus, and role-playing practice will help you with any eventuality you encounter. Even if something occurs that you had not considered at all, such as questions to which you do not know the answer, providing you keep your cool and have a clear idea of what is happening, you will be fine.

Taking a Celtic Reiki Workshop

When the time comes to start taking classes, practical preparation is often the best way to ensure success. Organising enough pens, paper, treatment couches, etc. is always essential, along with additional items, including name labels, drinking water, etc. The less you have to think about on the day the better, so ensure that you have prepared everything well in advance, so that nearer the time you can spend time on preparing yourself, rather than the class.

One excellent way of supporting yourself is to write cue cards, these contain short notes pertaining to each element of the workshop. They can be placed on your clipboard discreetly and read whilst students are doing their exercises, to minimise interference. These cards can contain each topic you want to cover in that session, with examples, and perhaps the main elements of each technique.

In the later iterations of the Celtic Reiki Master course we investigate 'Tree Plans', which are creative ways of systemising information into a highly memorable format. You can use a Tree Plan to map out foundation concepts, random thoughts and inspirations and supporting or structuring information. When planning and teaching your seminars, Tree Plans are highly recommended!

Some people like to write an entire script to memorise; yet this technique is cumbersome and relies entirely on one's memory abilities! It is often a better option to stick to role-play and rehearsal, thus developing your own, spontaneous style. Very often you will find that your 'Teacher Facet' comes to the forefront in a class, and you will undergo a metamorphosis as soon as you start to teach.

Of course, if you are having difficulty with the teaching processes, it is advisable to seek further training, particularly in teaching your target group.

Aftercare and Support

One of the most important roles you can have as a Master Teacher is that of a practitioner! As you nurture and support your students through the journey of self-development and confronting their past, you will employ your therapeutic skills in ensuring that the path is less bumpy and takes them where they are going at a quicker pace.

You cannot do the clearing, or healing for your students, as this is something they can only do for themselves, however, you can offer them a listening ear, or a sanctuary where they can ask any questions they might have, even after the course. Some students may make use of this aftercare, far more than others, but the important thing to consider is how much time you wish to commit to supporting your students.

Some teachers over-commit to caring for their students and create a co-dependent relationship. In these circumstances, it is possible for a teacher to become overworked, without sufficient time taken for themselves and their family, friends, etc.

As your students may require support after the course has been completed, a good understanding from the outset of what level of support you wish to provide is essential. Many Celtic Reiki teachers offer refresher, or workshop days as part of their course, so that students can return and ask questions, try the exercises they may not have used, and generally have a fun day.

There are also Masters who prefer to offer aftercare on a one-to-one basis. When doing this, is advisable to set boundaries, such as availability and hours in which it is appropriate for students to contact you. Many of these elements will already be in place from your professional practice.

Other Considerations

In addition to taking a course, or workshop, there are other factors that you should be aware of when teaching. Insurance, legal aspects, and marketing, etc. are all crucial to your planning and with every country having different regulations and laws, it is vital that you check what these are in your particular country of residence. It is also important that when working with groups, you always operate within the law and ensure that you are protected, as well as your students. Many of these subjects are included in Celtic Reiki Seminars or workshops that cover advice for small businesses or therapists.

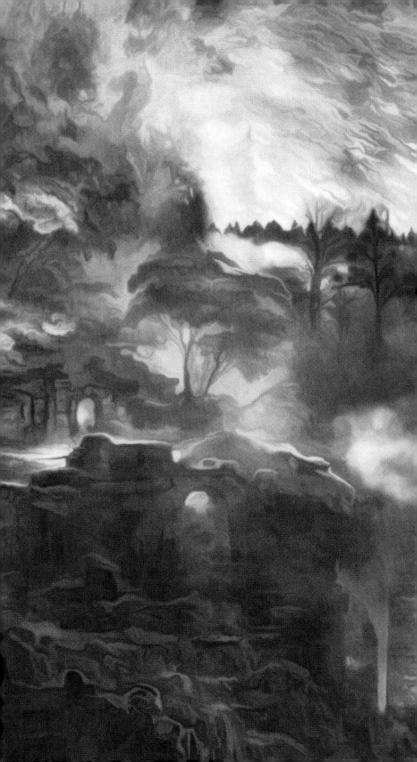

THE ART OF ESSENCE CREATION

We live in a Universe in which, absolutely everything, including physical matter is created from energy at a foundation level. The forces that drive our physical world interact to create solidity, which scientists now believe is the reason light, for example, travels in waves and interacts as particles of matter. When we look at the First Law of Thermodynamics, we see that energy cannot be created or destroyed – it only changes form; therefore the energy that creates solid materials does not suddenly disappear, eradicated in the process: it changes form, transforming to a different type of energy.

This can be deceptive as tables, trees, buildings, people, and so on, do not look or act like energy and therefore, in our human perspective, we forget that they are. The fact that solid objects do not shift and behave in a fluid way, such as light or heat, misleads our perception into believing they are somehow dissimilar to other forms of energy.

The Universe in which we live is infinite—it cannot

be quantified. Every single thing in existence creates the Universe and that is a lot of 'stuff'! In fact our Universe has no end and nothing can exist outside of it. For something to be outside the Universe, it must exist and if it exists, it is, in actuality inside the Universe. The thing we can glean from this is that everything that has ever happened in the Universe must be contained within it. We could say that all past events exist and must, therefore, exist in the Universe.

The reason this can be a challenge to comprehend is because we are so used to the notions of time and space; time being that moment then, to this moment now and space being that point here to that point over there. In our linear mindset, we look at things from moment to moment, place to place, forgetting that all things are one thing – all that exists is the Universe and the Universe is of all things that exist! If everything that has ever existed is contained within the Universe, it follows that everything that ever will happen also exists in the Universe. All possible outcomes and future events are right here, right now, we just have not perceived them yet.

From the idea of all things that exist on the material layers of perception are created from the interaction of energy, we understand each object or 'entity' having its own specific range of frequencies at an integral level. In other words, every individual organism and physical object possesses a unique range of vibrations that have an effect on the other vibrations it comes into contact with.

This immediately provides us with a challenge, because all energy is connected at an innate level, so where does the energy of one physical entity end and the another begin? Am I a separate, individual and autonomous being or are the points where I become something else and something else becomes me? These questions are not ones that many people ponder, in fact most people have quite a clear idea of who they are – certainly if the occurrence of the words 'I', 'mine', 'my' and 'me' are anything to go by! However, when creating an energy therapy to say that a range of vibrations are 'this energy' and not 'that energy' suggests separation and fragmentation.

To counteract this internalised divorcing of energy, I decided that Celtic Reiki would use the concept of an 'essence'. Not necessarily a specific 'range' or 'band' of vibrations, but vibrations of energy from a particular perspective. Thus, the inherent nature of every essence is that all things are perceived, using single point or perspective. The Ioho Essence is the Universe viewed from the perspective of Yew Trees, whilst the Saille Essence is that of the Willow. You could also say that your Essence is all energy, connected to and viewed from your unique viewpoint of the Universe.

As you expand your awareness of the vibrational realms, you integrate new perspectives into your consciousness and therefore create a new outlook. The more you understand the world at a vibrational level, the more you learn about how to create holistic health and well-being using different essences. With each new encounter, you integrate energetically and physically the knowledge of individual plants, animals, minerals, etc. gaining new insights and unique perspectives on all levels.

Even though, in Celtic Reiki, we focus on the natural world and in particular trees, we can go beyond the realms of the physical world and see how types of energy, such as radiation, visible light and sound can be used therapeutically. We can also use the energy of concepts, such as time, space, even mythical animals and iconography. When we examine as many vibrations as our journey and imagination will permit, we create an extensive range of perspectives that are entrained to work in a therapeutic environment and by doing so, we not only benefit our client's holistic health, but our own.

Now, although it often perceived as an 'energy therapy', in the same umbrella as Usui Reiki practices, Celtic Reiki actually integrates two distinct categories of complementary therapy. These are: 'Therapeutic Entrainment' and 'Vibrational Medicine'. Examples of

Entrainment Therapies include Usui Reiki, Binaural Therapy and Therapeutic Touch, whilst Vibrational Medicines encompass Homoeopathy, Colour Therapy, Flower Essences, etc. This amazing synthesis gives the treatment ease of Therapeutic Entrainment and the incredible range of Homoeopathy combined into a single powerful and wide reaching practice.

Working completely energetically, the Celtic Reiki Master harvests and defines energy in the form of essences from trees, the world around them and, indeed further a-field. These essences are catalogued, stored and tested, before being used in a professional therapeutic environment. The vibrations are applied by the therapist, either as a single essence, or in combination, to the client via an entrainment process.

Practitioners of vibrational medicines use a variety of physical implements to administer the vibrations depending on the therapy in question. Homoeopaths use pharmaceutically prepared remedies, which are created from a substance or vibration and often supplied in liquid or tablet form. These are given to the client to be self-administered at specific times. Essences, such as Bach's Flower Remedies, are created from vibrations that are stored in water and preserved in alcohol. Machines are also used in Colour, Sound, Magnetic and Light Therapies.

Celtic Reiki Essences are harvested and stored energetically (as carefully, specifically defined memories/ unconscious parameters) and then prescribed by the therapist or master via a process of therapeutic entrainment; this alleviates the requirement of equipment or substances. Therefore, there are many advantages over the traditionally used techniques, as this method increases the range and application of existing energy therapies, whilst negating the need for expensive equipment or storage space, etc.

The adaptability, flexibility and expansive nature of harvesting new essences makes Celtic Reiki an extremely powerful and fulfilling therapy once it has been mastered.

With practice and a little commitment, it can become a rewarding profession and fascinating learning experience that will help improve your health, as well as that of the people you treat.

In my book "The Official Guide to Karmic Regression Therapy and Karmic Reiki" (mPowr), there is an in-depth exploration of traditional energy systems and the physiology of our energy 'senses'. This vibrational anatomy is very relevant here and provides us with an understanding of how we translate the Universe at a vibrational level into sensory information, thoughts, actions and physical results.

In the harvesting, collecting and application of Celtic Reiki Essences, we require the use of what are known as the 'Peri- Systems' (see Oschman) to sense, recognise, remember and emulate the frequencies of energy we employ. These Peri- Systems are dense accumulations of connective tissue that surround and encase various systems of the body, namely: the nerves (Perineural), muscles (Perimysial), bones (Periosteal), and blood vessels (Perivascular). These systems are believed to be responsible for the communication of vibrations throughout the body. This process happens naturally in our everyday lives, usually for the coordination of healing injury, among other things. Nevertheless, to achieve conscious awareness of the vibrations that flow through our Peri- Systems, particulatly for professional entrainment, we can use some specific points of the body and various exercises to help us.

Originated from the traditions of particular Eastern practices, combined with contemporary techniques, we acquire the capacity to strengthen our energy system and increase our conscious sensitivity to the energy vibrations we encounter.

The Eastern way of describing the Perineural System is via a system of meridians that run from the tips of our toes and fingers to the head, thus extending the entire length of our body. All of these meridians pass through a point in the abdomen, known as the Dantien. There is a distinct analogy between the meridian logic and the Perineural System, which can often be more useful in practical application. So, we shall use this concept to describe the important areas of our anatomy, used when working with Celtic Reiki, because of our Eastern connections in philosophy.

Throughout the meridian systems are many pressure points, some of which create real value for us in Celtic Reiki. The CV1/GV1 point is located at the Perineum, between the anus and genitals. The GV28 is located at the roof of the mouth and the CV24 on the tip of the tongue; by placing the tongue to the roof of the mouth, just behind the teeth, a bond between these two points is created.

The Dantien is seen in Eastern therapies such as Shiatsu and Reiki as the centre of energy, a little like a giant energy 'store' that can be cultivated and developed. By doing this, a practitioner/client can increase their natural ki (or chi) connection and thus create holistic health. This is similar to the idea of raising vibrations to a higher level and thus increasing the energy in the vibrations of our Peri- Systems.

The Practitioner and Master of Celtic Reiki creates conscious changes in their body's energy system to conduct a range of predetermined essences and projects these through a connection to their client, subject or focus. These essences are reproduced in accordance with the Practitioner's perspective. The client or subject will, in turn, entrain their own energy systems to evoke a change at a molecular level.

This creates a change in the client's perspective of health, development and wellbeing as they translate the essences into their own perception of the vibrations. The Practitioner's perspective then alters to encompass this adjusted view of the original essence and the two parties gradually balance the frequencies of energy between them, until they are both resonating at the same rate or from a mutual perspective.

The outcome of this is that the client has learnt new essences at a molecular level, initiating a healing process and the practitioner has enhanced and refined their knowledge of the specific essences used in the treatment, as a result, gaining a multidimensional view of the vibration and its uses. This 'energetic communication' and discovery has the overall effect of 'raising your vibrations', which basically means that the general effect of a treatment is to increase the frequency of electromagnetic energy associated with your body and holistic being - the higher the frequency of your vibrations then the more energy is contained within.

Every person, every living thing is unique and totally unlike any other. Our individual expression of perspective is unlike any other and in a Universe that is energy the expression of perspective as experienced through separateness is a novel concept. Imagine a Universe that knows absolutely everything about itself (hence, it knows absolutely everything), except what it is to not know about itself. In our disconnection from the Universe, we are experiencing something that the Universe as a whole has never encountered – what it is like not to be all-knowing: what it is to be cut off and alone. This parallel with Shinki, underlies our Celtic Reiki philosophy of Ki.

Each of us feels this loneliness at birth, as we are thrust in a cold, clinical world, wrenched from connection, bound by a strange, restricting, uncomfortable body. From the moment of our birth, we seek reconnection. We know this at a fundamental level but, as separate beings, this knowledge is filtered through our concept of detachment and isolation. So we fall in love; we make friendships and find partners. Sometimes these bonds last a lifetime, sometimes they are broken and we run the risk of getting hurt. We might also choose other forms of connection, such as an affinity with animals, or the environment, or money, or work, or music, or creativity. We are always expressing our need for unity but do this through unique natures and so relate to the physical world in the way that only we can.

As children, we are very aware of our energetic nature and are very intuitive in our outlook. It is not long, however, before the physical teachings and limited beliefs are installed and we lose our energy sense. Each time we are told a limiting belief, we are offered a statement with a particular dynamic, which often cause us to contract further into isolation and the illusion of separateness.

When we are contracted in perspective and limited in perception, the overall vibration of our Peri- Systems lessens, thus lowering our vitality. We may begin to experience fear, anger, hate, jealousy, sadness and so on, until in our adulthood we also are saturated with worry, stress, anxiety, and many other contractive emotions. These are the sorts of traumas that weigh us down and create mental/emotional/physical illness, starving us of happiness and making us feel even more alone and hurt.

We can choose to stay connected to these contractive dynamics, completely bogged down by a victim's outlook of the world, until the day we return to our original source. Sometimes though, something miraculous occurs and we begin to realise there is more to life than we have been led to believe and we begin to expand our dynamics and revitalise our vibrations, actively working towards a higher perspective of ourselves and our lives. This can be done through creativity, sports, work, therapy, love and so on. As we lift our energy, we shake free of the old views and become happier and more 'connected' once again.

Celtic Reiki offers an adaptable system to speed up and support this process, enabling an accelerated voyage to health, well-being and happiness on all levels; initially, by the Practitioner working with prescribed (Orientated/Calibrated) essences, then as a Master by harvesting and using a range of new essences. This procedure is then enhanced and propagated by the use of these vibrations in a therapeutic environment.

With the knowledge that every time you conduct a treatment, you gain a new perspective on the essences you use. By a gradual balancing out of your vibrations with those of your client, you gain a greater comprehension of the perspectives that you are consciously aware of.

It is usually at this point the question arises that if you are treating somebody with a severe energy trauma and you start to 'take on' their energy, is this safe? There is one golden rule to remember at all times in Celtic Reiki: "Energy is energy, is energy!"

Confusion often arises when we are working with essences in a physical environment as Practitioners sometimes confuse the balancing of vibrations with the root causes of disease and trauma. If you are treating Mrs X, for example, who had a terribly traumatic childhood, you are in no danger of taking on that trauma. As you treat Mrs X with various essences, you gain a new perspective of the essences you are using, by experiencing the vibration through Mrs X's perspective. There is no 'taking on' of energy, or 'release of trauma', you are simply changing energy from one form to another and then learning the new energy vibration that has been created. No energy is negative energy; only the connotations we attach to the energy are negative.

All things have a vibration; an energy frequency and in creating your Celtic Reiki Essences, you will learn how to 'remember' and use these in a therapeutic environment. This process can be done without any sensory awareness of the vibrations in question, as your unconscious mind will know how these processes are done.

You may discover that in the first stages of practice you actually feel very little or nothing and this can be the case, especially if you only have a limited amount of experience or are new to working with energy on a conscious level. I am certain you want to sense the diversity in sensation of the assorted vibrations you come into contact with and thus, you will want to get to the point where Celtic Reiki is a sumptuously perceptive and sensual experience.

This process may happen instantly and naturally for a lot of people. If it does not happen for you, do not worry – it is comparable with going to the gym: at first the Peri-Systems are sluggish and weak, atrophied from lack of use. As you exercise the various systems, you strengthen them and they can cope with more energy, more vibrations, more information. The greater the focus you place on sensory information from your Peri- Systems, the easier you will find it to sense the vibrations in finer detail.

This is not in the hands of fate, or chance, nor is it different for everybody except you. It is physiology, plain and simple. Yes, some people can develop muscle mass faster than others, some can metabolise food quicker, but the fact is that with practice, trust and confidence, you will experience the data from your Peri- senses.

Preparing to Harvest

Before a Celtic Reiki Master begins the Harvesting process, I recommend that they spend some time preparing some form of structure of framework for their Essences. Some Masters have created their own catalogue of literally hundreds of Essences, not only of Trees, Plants and Minerals, but of all forms of perspective. Creating a good system of categorisation can not only assist you in keeping track of and having easy recall of Essences, it can help you to understand each Essence better, through the detailed listing of your Harvest, testing and Application feedback.

To support new Harvesters, I suggest the following method of categorisation, with the recommendation that you adapt this to your own needs and personal preferences. With an infinite range of vibrations to choose from, the use of simple categories can provide a greater ease of use generically. As you explore your own Harvesting habits, you may find you require additional categories or extra detail in one particular category. For example, you may want to divide

Trees into sub-categories or distinguish different Essences by cultural connections, perspectives, and so on (Oak, Duir, Quercus Robur, etc.)

The definition of an essence is equally as important (if not more so) than the energetic vibrations. This is because definition is what gives energy, physical form and grounding. Time and money are both formed of infinite energy, but their definition is finite and it is this that makes time and money so important to many people. The more complex the definition you provide for a new essence, the greater refinement in results you will achieve - for instance: an essence that helps ease arthritic pain in the metacarpals of the left hand will be more effective when treating that dis-ease than an essence for 'arthritis' would on the same issue. Do remember that heightened detail in your essences will also create the need for more essences!

To start the process, I sort essences into a series of Archetypes, for which I have defined corresponding 'Harvest Essences' for use by Celtic Reiki Masters when harvesting. The Archetypes are: Trees/Plants, Animals, Minerals, Microscopic, Artificial, Energy, Places, Concepts, Additional.

Suggested Essence Archetypes

Trees and Other Plants

The Trees and Other Plants category includes all vegetation, including fruits, seeds, nuts, etc. and fungi, lichen, algae, etc. If you wish to work extensively with plant matter, you may decide to add sub-classifications, such as: evergreens, shrubs, vegetables, and so on.

Animals

Animals include mammals, reptiles, fish and insects and whilst you may decide to place any animal in the section, there might be some you encounter that are so small you decide to use 'Microscopic' instead. Once again, you may require sub-categories if you intend to work with animals the majority of the time, or in the on-going creation of your therapy.

Minerals

Minerals can be a wide-ranging classification, from all rocks, crystals and metals, to liquids such as water, gases such as neon and more complex minerals, such as plasmas, etc. It is strongly advised that in this category, you create sub-divisions.

Microscopic

This interesting category encompasses all minute particles, both living and non-living. These can include bacteria, viruses, parasites, and so forth, until you reach sub-atomic particles and other quanta.

Artificial

This vast classification covers anything that has been artificially created from plastics and fibres, through to chemical products, and even machines and buildings. As well as the category with most scope, it can also be the one that creates the most indecision, for example, if you are harvesting the vibration of 'music', you might want this to go into Artificial, or it could go into Energy. A substance, such as 'Quorn' could be a Plant, but as it is a 'cultured fungus' it could easily fit in Artificial as well; the decision is completely yours.

Energy

Light, sound, radiation, and so on all comprise this classification, which can also include other energy therapy vibrations, such as the energy of Seichim, or Usui Reiki, etc. This is also a good place to store the energy created by movement (waterfall, wind, tide, etc.)

Places

Places can be seen as an extension of both Artificial and Energy, as the Master is harvesting the vibration of a physical, or energetic place. Places could encompass examples such as, Stonehenge, London, The Moon, Sirius (Star), and so on.

Concepts

These are things that are not necessarily physical, but are nevertheless imaginable. So for this category you could harvest, the energy of a book, or song, maybe a mystical beast such as a Unicorn, or Phoenix, you might choose the energy of a significant date, time, or of concepts such as a 'Hypercube', 'Chaos', 'Inner Child', etc.

Additional

This classification has a dual purpose, firstly for substances that do not fit, or fit into too many of the other categories; an illustration of this could be the vibration of the homoeopathic remedy 'Dolphin', which is not made from a Dolphin, but contains a group dynamic, meditating on the concept of a Dolphin (Energy, Concept, Animal, Artificial, Mineral).

The second use for this category is for combined essences that you trigger on a regular basis, so have created a new single essence for ease of use. An example of this is when you combine the birthstone, ruling planet, metal and the colour of a particular zodiac sign and use the combined essences to treat a person of that sign. (Venus, Opal, Blue, Copper, combined could be called 'Libra').

Organisation of the Essences

When classifying objects, you will discover the method of cataloguing vibrations that best suits you and the way you work. To help you with this, the following section is dedicated to offering examples and tips on how to go about creating the tools with which you intend to work. The current situation in the United States means that keeping clear and precise records about harvests and essence is a worthwhile practice and this will surely be the case in other countries in the future. With this in mind, I recommend the first three types of record keeping. Whatever means you eventually decide to use, remember the one golden piece of advice. Good organisation will make your practice a whole lot easier!

Books & Manuals

This is probably the simplest method for recording information on each essence that you harvest. Some people decide to use a notebook and write down the development of each essence as it happens. Depending on how you work, you may require a single book, one for each Archetype, or even one for each essence! When appropriate, you could transfer your written notes to a typed format and have these printed.

You may decide to type the information directly using a Word Processor, or other form of computerised data storage, however be aware that it is always wise to have a small notebook a hand, as you never know when new information will come through!

Reference Cards

As above, instead, using postcard size cards to write the main points of each essence and some background information. This is an excellent way of having a concise, alphabetical record of essences in your treatment environment, as quick reminder or cross-reference. Even if you decide to use another method of classification, this is still a good idea, especially if you have a tendency to forget essences, or have an extensive range of essences in your catalogue.

Databases (Spreadsheets, etc.)

A computerised database is, undoubtedly, the most efficient way of managing the classification process, albeit the most technical. By using a software package to input all the information you glean for each essence, you can not only prescribe quickly and proficiently, but you can also cross reference and keep an ongoing record of your client's treatment programme and progress.

The downside of this method is, of course, technical knowhow, yet there are plenty of workshops and courses that can teach you how to computerise your practice. Another consideration here is whether you want a computer in your therapeutic environment and the effect this will have on the room, holistically.

Crystals

The last two methods are only advised if you are an experienced energy worker and have a lot of confidence! I would also ask that you research the laws of your country to ascertain what type of record (if any) is required of the treatments and essences you use. Crystals do retain a huge amount of information vibrationally, can be cross-referenced and used as prescribing tools.

You can encode the information, using the crystal as a trigger (as you would use a Kotodama or symbol). This is a process in which you can attach energy, using the crystal as a 'hook' – the crystal does not retain the energy, but it will act as a reminder when you activate the essence.

Purely Energetically

This is an approach that means you do not keep written notes, but instead work completely energetically; an energetic equivalent to the oral tradition! You simply trust that the essences will be remembered; you will intuit the prescription and your body will remember the correct frequency to reproduce. To a certain extent, this process is involved in Celtic Reiki all the time, but if you are confident, it is possible for you to work without hooks and labels, thus forgoing any physical attachment.

TOOLS FOR THE HARVEST

Once you have taken the decision to begin creating your own essences, I would recommend two tools that will help you prepare for your first harvests. The Celts and other indigenous people throughout history are reputed to have a very close connection to the Earth; sensing minute shifts in vibration, weather patterns, and other dynamics of their surrounding environment. In modern cultures and particular in and around the big cities of the Western world we have lost this connection to a major extent.

Housed within buildings of brick, concrete, glass, and wood, we are likely to have water and heat piped into our homes and have become completely dependent on electricity for most of our needs. Immersed in electromagnetic fields and without needing to be aware of the world around us, we have a tendency to be divorced from our Earth. Most people do not know which way is north, how to start a fire without artificial means of ignition, and where to find the nearest, natural supply of fresh water – one of our most basic needs.

In addition to our disconnection from our own planet, is the distance we often create from our own inner-self. We tend to lead such stressful lives that our heads are usually in a frantic state of highly awakened focus. This is wonderful when thinking hard, dealing with a busy day, doing some form of physical activity, or being 'on the ball', but when we want creativity, connection and a wakeful state of peace and serenity, it's not so good.

The first technique listed here can help us to restore a natural connection to the world, through adjusting our own vibrations to match the resonance of the Earth. The second tool changes our brain state to a more relaxed, creative and aware attitude that helps us connect to our inner-senses and vibrational focus. These can both be used on an ongoing basis to maintain a powerful connection to the Earth, the natural world, and the other hotspots on your harvest adventures!

The Schumann Resonance

The Schumann Resonance is a natural phenomenon which is created by the sum of all lightning around the globe. The electromagnetic pulses created by lightning bounces between the Earth's surface and the ionosphere, creating a frequency of between 1 and 40Hz. The exact frequency fluctuates depending on the global thunderstorm activity, local meteorological conditions and conductivity of the Earth's surface, in conjunction with lunar position, Sun spots and so on.

When you bring your perspective in alignment with the Schumann Resonance at any given time, you provide your energy work with richer degree of harmony. If you activate this frequency of energy each day and send the vibration throughout your physical body, you can adjust yourself to the current resonance of the Earth (a continually fluctuating factor!). By doing this, you will be exercising your energy systems, adjusting your overall energy to the earth, thus creating a very strong connection to the planet and enhancing your sensitivity abilities accordingly.

Many of the Masters I have worked with, who activate the Schumann Resonance regularly, describe an array of beneficial incentives for regulating your Peri-systems with those of the Earth on a daily basis. These testimonials accredit the Schumann Resonance with greater sensation and sensitivity in practice, greater awareness and connection with the planet and environment, feeling of peace, serenity and even motivation, as well as a host of other amazing results.

On a Celtic Reiki Master Programme, you'll learn how to trigger the Schumann Essence. You will then be guided to work through breathing in a specific way and use your meridian system to create a profound connection to the resonance. This is the foundation for your harvesting and testing of Essences, as well as a fabulous addition to therapy and developmental practices.

Alpha Rhythm

The electromagnetic energy emitted by the brain can be categorised depending the frequency of the brainwaves. These different 'rhythms' place us into specific 'brain-states' depending upon the Hertz measurement of the rhythm. The four main brain-states are classified as Beta, Alpha, Theta, and Delta (there are also Epsilon, Gamma and Lambda states, though these tend to be rarer).

- Beta 14-50Hz – Wide-awake
- Alpha 8-14Hz – Very relaxed, heightened creativity
- Theta 4-7 Hz – Meditation, or light sleep
- Delta 1/3-4Hz – Deep Sleep, or unconsciousness

By entering the brain-state known as Alpha Rhythm, we consciously access parts of our mind that may not be familiar with in usual waking consciousness, particularly if you have a tendency to be quite stressed or have a busy lifestyle. By readdressing any deficiency of time spent in Alpha Rhythm, we create a strong link between these and our conscious mind. This process could be equated to a light meditative state, in which the subject is awake and yet very relaxed. In addition to assisting us in the sensing of essences, this magical state can help improve memory, intuitive response and creative impulse.

In order to sense and interpret the variation in energy frequencies, we rely on information provided to the brain by the numerous Peri- Systems via the Ascending Reticular Activating System. The ARAS is responsible for consciousness and can be viewed as a filter through which all sensory data passes. It is the Reticular System that points your consciousness to important information. As this process is programmed and habitual, we need a way of instruct the ARAS that the data sent from the Peri- systems is of importance to us. In the Orientation and Calibration process of Celtic Reiki mastership your ARAS begins to alter its criteria; working in Alpha Rhythm can also help you to shift the focus and gain a greater degree of information from the Peri- systems.

You may also find it easier to intensify the link between conscious recognition of essences and unconscious interpretation of their unique perspective, by entering the Alpha State, using this wonderful technique created by Jose Silva and listed in his book The Silva Method.

Technique:

Sit in a comfortable chair, where you will not be disturbed for a few minutes and close your eyes. With your eyes remaining closed, look up and 20 degrees to the right, as if staring at a clock face and looking to "1 o'clock". Hold this eye position as you count down from 100 to 1 in your head, each number counted with a 2 second gap left in between. When you finish this exercise you will be in Alpha State!

Harvesting Essences

One of the first things you will need to keep in mind when creating your range of Celtic Reiki Essences is that harvesting is a very personal process. The type and amount of essences you start with, how you record these and what plans you make for on-going harvesting and testing are all factors to consider.

The energetic process is two-tiered and uses two distinct essences; the first being a 'Universal Harvest Essence' and the second is dependent on the Archetypal classification of the essence you wish to harvest. These Harvest Essences have associated symbols and mantras which you will learn all about on your Celtic Reiki Experience.

A Brief word on Contraindications

In all therapies, we need to be aware of any possible contraindications, as a consequence of what we are doing with regards to our client, so if we are working with a client who is pregnant, or uses a pacemaker, has a shunt fitted, is hypertensive, and so on, we know how to adapt our treatment method to ensure our client's well-being.

Even though energy therapies are very gentle in nature, they can be powerful in action, so you should be aware that even in situations where detoxification is induced through treatment, this is a positive and health-inspiring state. Thus Celtic Reiki does not cause harm and is completely safe to use. When it comes to harvesting, however, you need to be aware of contraindications such as the toxicity of some plants, the unpredictable nature of some animals, harmful minerals, and so on. Therefore, do be absolutely sure of the nature of what you are harvesting and act appropriately when conducting any activity that brings you into contact with a substance, living creature, etc.

The Harvest Begins!

The first frequency of energy that we use in both the collection of vibrations and in a treatment is that of the Universal Harvest Essence. In the first stages of practice you activate this essence before you proceed, although you may find it activates automatically, negating the need for intentional triggering. The Mastership or Advanced Master Orientation that you Calibrate to towards the end of your course will be accompanied with information on what this essence is and how to work with it.

When employed in the harvesting of vibrations, Universal Harvest Essence basically filters out any 'background noise' in an energetic sense. Creating a clarity and purity to your essences that will be of benefit during testing and application. By adjusting to the level of the UHE, you are basically 'wiping the energetic slate' so that you and your harvest subject are on the same energetic level and you gain an accurate sense of the vibrations you're connecting to.

Therefore the UHE is an excellent essence to invoke whenever a clearer picture of the surrounding environment is needed. For example, the essence can also be applied outside of a treatment, or harvesting environment whenever there are feelings of unease, depression, or anger and so on, caused by being 'out of sync'. By triggering the essence you can have a soothing effect on yourself, your surrounding environment and the people in it.

Harvesting the Universe

Anything that has vibration can be harvested, no matter how high, or low the frequency. This means that everything can be harvested, because everything is energy! A single thought, or an entire ocean can be harvested; a slight breeze, or the brightest star, there is no vibration that is inaccessible to the Celtic Reiki Master, although it may take practice to actually recognise some vibrations on a sensory level.

I view an essence as the entire Universe from a single perspective. This means that 'your essence' would be the entire Universe viewed through your entire sensory experience of it – not only at this moment, but every moment you have and will have experienced. When we physically perceive essences, however, we do so physically, through our senses and this translates to an experience in space and time. Thus, essences are often sensed as waves of energy, or vibrations that can be felt directly or via synaesthesia.

These vibrations exist in every single thing, however some of the types of energy you may wish to harvest will have a complex range of frequencies, to get an accurate picture of this essence, every frequency will need collection and remembering. This often takes practice, but do not let that stop you, over time you can re-harvest the essence and add any new information to the existing image you have. This creates essences that are multifaceted (such as the individual trees of a Celtic Essence and the species the tree is a part of) and therefore have many features and a much greater efficiency in the treatment environment.

The harvesting procedure can be as easy as you want it to be: essences are made, simply by consciously recognising and remembering a particular set of vibrations. Many do prefer to have some form of routine that helps to focus intent and it is certainly advisable to do this in the majority of instances. Over time, you will certainly find that you evolve your personal and unique way of collecting.

Each of the Archetypal Harvest Essences has a particular perspective, ideally suited to its own form of essence source. In definition, they have no effect on the finished Celtic Reiki Essence, other than creating an ease of use and clarity that makes your role as the harvester much more enjoyable. After extensive use in the field the nuances of each different essence have been revealed. Consequently, each essence has been assigned an Archetypal classification, yet you may decide to use these creatively, for example if harvesting the vibration of your pet cat, you may wish to use the 'Concept Essence' to collect the qualities of the cat species, rather than using the 'Animal Archetype' to harvest the exact essence of your individual feline! Alternatively, you could use the 'Animal Essence' on the concept of a Dragon in order to highlight the animalistic qualities of the creature.

Trees and Plants

When you come to harvest a plant in any form, the first thing you should bear in mind, is to inform the plant, tree, etc. what you intend to do, re-assure the plant that you will not harm him and ask his permission. These steps are in fact the most important activity in the whole procedure of harvesting plant vibrations. Over the years of originating Celtic Reiki I have come to consider plant-life with exactly the same respect as you would another person. Trees and shrubs have been treated with little, or no respect since the disappearance of the Celtic peoples and after centuries of being regarded as 'things', many of the wisest plant-folk have become deeply mistrusting and suspicious of humankind.

Through intimate dealings with these wonderful creatures, I have learnt just how important it is to realise the intricate balance that exists between plant and animal species. In a physical sense we feel superior, as we can move and talk and create things, although energetically trees and plants are just as conscious as we are. Certainly with the older trees, they are wiser and more knowledgeable about life, too.

By treating each plant as an equal, rather than something to possess and take from, we develop a global relationship with our plant cousins. We can learn from them, as they learn from us and we share our perspective and knowledge, rather than entering into what could be called an abusive relationship.

Each time we deal with a plant, our natural perspective is altered and we vibrationally display that alteration to every plant we encounter subsequently. If you harvest a frequency from a plant, without asking, it may affect future harvesting, as the plants you encounter may resist, or alter their perception in reaction to 'just another human' who disrespects them. However, by ensuring that you communicate your intent and ask permission, the plant will offer gladly and you will have made a friend for life!

This ethic is one that is at the spiritual heart of Celtic

Reiki, which is about loving all things and being in complete harmony with the world around us. So when you propose to harvest the essence of a tree, even though you are not taking anything from the tree, you should ask his permission first. The energy you sense and re-create in your Peri- systems has not been removed from anywhere and you have not been given anything. By acknowledging the tree, however, you have given respect to the tree and this is the key – by offering the tree something and not expecting anything in return the worst that can happen is the need to go and find another tree! What can happen is that the tree will offer you something back and this can be the most magical of all experiences.

Once you have obtained the goodwill of the plant in question, centre yourself and activate the UHE, followed by the Plant Archetypal Essence (either by using the appropriate triggers or from memory). The essence that is best suited to plants is one of very intense focus, as this converges right in the heart of the plant and centres your perspective at the very essence of his being. As you do this, you may feel a pressure or energy sensation (such as vibrations, heat, cold, etc.) emanating back out at you – this is the energy signature integrating with your bioenergetic field. If you do not feel this, do not worry, just stick with the process, knowing that it is working.

As you continue, the energy should get stronger and begin to centre on your hands, feet, or maybe in the lower abdomen. You can help the progression of the harvest by allowing the energy to pervade your energy field – being open to it – and if necessary permitting it to move you (some people report a pulling back, or spiralling motion, others may find their hands being pushed further apart, or a turning of their head). Always stay grounded if this happens to avoid falling over!

This is the point where you attach your own essence trigger, if required, by attaching a name, or similar 'label' to the essence. This is the trigger you will use later in prescription and treatment situations. If you are using a notebook, write down the trigger as soon as you have completed the harvest.

You should be aware when your physiology has integrated the essence, either through a feeling of restlessness, or of 'letting go', or just a sense that it has been done. At this point, thank the plant and wish him well. You may like to offer some Celtic Reiki and if it does want to experience this, you will feel as if you are being held, magnetically pulled in, or maybe stuck to the ground, etc.

Remember to make notes, including the time, date, plant type and any intuitive information, or sensory effects you had during the harvest.

Animals

As with plants, you should always maintain a respect for your animal subject, explain what you are doing and ask permission. Do bear in mind that animals react differently to plants and, whilst animals do tend to be more aware of energy that humans, their sensitivity is not as refined as that of plant species. So be prepared for the animal to run off or recoil when you start the harvest process.

Celtic Reiki cannot harm any living thing; conversely by using it, you may actually promote a healing environment for the subject, so harvesting is good for them. Without prior experience of the sensations, however, animals may just be uncertain of what is happening and prefer to retreat. You should be aware, when dealing with larger animals, or those with teeth and claws that they may want to get 'through you' in order to get away! You should always be prepared for unpredictability when working with animals and it is perfectly acceptable to wear protective clothing where necessary. If you find certain animals just too daunting to harvest from, but still would like their vibration, you can also use 'Concept Essence' to harvest the perspective of the creature in question.

When harvesting vibrations from animals, there will be many different frequencies to deal with, as bones, blood vessels, muscles, etc. all vibrates at different rates. So decide before you start whether you wish to harvest the essence of the whole animal or a certain part; teeth, bone, blood, etc. A particularly useful vibration is unhealthy tissue, such as skin conditions, tumours, etc. as these can be used to help heal the issue on others.

Once you ask gained permission from your subject, trigger the Animal Archetypal Essence by intent, or by visualising the trigger in hands. Place your hands on both sides of the animal and project your focus inwards. The process should be very similar to that with plants, but allow for variations in strength and vibration. Animals tend to be hotter too!

When the harvest is underway, attach your trigger label and complete the essence collection, remembering always to thank the animal upon completion. Make your notes as usual, adding any intuitive, or sensory feedback from the harvest and any reactions from the subject (if you are harvesting from human subjects, ask for their feedback too).

Minerals

Minerals include such a vast range of subjects that each situation you encounter will call for a different technique and it is very much a case of taking each occurrence as it is presented to you. Common mineral essences you may wish to harvest are: crystals, metal, rock, water, etc. and we shall discuss these here.

When you are harvesting crystal vibrations, remember that you are working with a living entity and therefore should, once again, explain your intent and ask permission. Crystals have a definite way of responding and that is, if it does not hurt or burn, it's OK to proceed!

To harvest from Crystals, Metals and loose rock simply hold the subject in your hand, activate the Mineral Archetypal Essence. If you are harvesting from a huge amount of a mineral, for example a mountainside, beach, etc. just place your hands flat against the surface of the subject and project your intent deeply into the ground, visualising the vibrations splashing up, all around you. On the contrary, if you are dealing with a fragile, or minute mineral subject, such as a snowflake, or diamond fragment, simply place your hands over the subject and let the energy 'flit' around it.

Water is of special consideration, because it actually retains vibrations, like a vibrational memory. This is why some water is seen to be healing (Chalice Well, Lourdes, etc.) and why some can be detrimental to health (mineral, or radiation poisoning). Whenever you encounter a new source of water, I would advise you to create a new essence rather than mixing perspectives to the same label.

Microscopic

There are two types of microscopic vibrations you may wish to harvest; those from microbes, such as bacteria, amoeba, parasites, etc. or non-living, dust, and so forth. The Microscopic Archetypal Essence will work for both types of microscopic.

It is important to consider whether you ask permission from the microbes you are working with. Some Masters do not bother, especially with viral agents — yet the viral and bacterial agents do have a sort of collective consciousness or hive mind that you can communicate with, after some practice. I have discovered through experience that many a viral or bacterial consciousness will deny the harvest, so a way to gain access to microbes without seeking permission is to ascertain the availability of that microscopic as a homoeopathic remedy (many subjects can be found this way, in all categories). This is particularly useful with illnesses such as HIV/AIDS, Herpes, and so on, as these are readily available from a homoeopathic pharmacy. Be aware, however, that the process of 'potentisation' has prepared these remedies.

Trigger the Microscopic Archetypal Essence and pull the resulting sensations into your hands. Then, continue with the aforementioned harvest procedures.

Artificial

As with minerals, the Artificial class is so massive, that individual situations should be tackled as they arise. You will harvest the energy of mobile phone in a very different way from a jumbo jet! For that reason, I shall leave the method up to you, suffice to say that the Artificial Archetypal Essence is extremely versatile and will help you to harvest almost anything!

Energy

Energy forms one of the most fascinating Archetypes we, as therapists, can come into contact with. Homoeopathic remedies of radioactive materials, sound and various coloured lights have shown us that there is a huge amount of scope here, especially when dealing with many of the modern dis-eases and trauma that we encounter as complementary therapists.

As energy is so intangible, the best way to harvest a vibration is to visualise the essence moving slowly down to you and gradually passing down the length of your body. Then imagine the essence in question swirling around your body and being gathered up into your Peri- systems.

When writing your notes, remember to describe the details of how you conducted the harvest and any extra information that is available about the essence. "Fire vibration collected from log and coal fuelled fire..." "Light vibration from 60w tungsten bulb..." and so on.

Places

The essence of a place may seem a strange inclusion here, as energy does not know time, nor space and therefore, cannot recognise a 'place' as we do. However, places do have a perspective and can be seen as the physical labels for a specific perspective. Anybody who has experienced the healing peace of a church, or the invigoration of a cliff top, the atmosphere of a theatrical performance or a concert will appreciate, it is usually a mixture of environment, people (or lack of) and other living things, motion and so on that synthesise to create the ambience of a place. The Places Archetypal Essence is similar to the previous essence; however it is more focused on what we would perceive to be the surrounding physical area.

The Places Essence also relates to areas of space, such as stars, or planets and places in time, so you can harvest the vibrations of historical events, such as the energy of a battlefield to help those traumatised by war, etc.

When harvesting the essence of a place, you should, wherever possible, include in your notes, information about the time and date, geographic location and you may find it help to make notes about the weather conditions, physical situation (people around and so forth), plus other physical factors that may have affected the energy.

Concepts

The Concept Archetypal Essence is the most fascinating, when working on the harvesting of imagery, mythology, or belief. Basically you have free reign to include whatever you like in your definition of the resulting essence, from Dragons and Unicorns, to a favourite passage from a Holy Book, or song. You can work with art forms, mathematical theories, dreams and anything else that has been imagined, believed, or conceptualised in some way.

Whenever you are working with a concept, especially one that has a 'living form', such as a mythological beast, Deity, Angel, Faerie and so on, do remember to treat the concept as a living being. For in some place, be it called another dimension, or parallel reality, this creature does exist! So be sure to explain your intent, ask permission and say thank you.

In the note writing of these harvest sessions, but sure to include information on any images, or physical hooks used to connect into the conceptual energy. Such as, "Listened to the CD." "Stared at the picture of..." "Meditated on the thought of..."

Additional

When working with miscellaneous essences, it will reside with your personal judgment, which essence to use, depending on the entity, object or energy that you are harvesting. You may decide to use the trigger nearest to the subject matter or just to use intent, in which case, you may find the UHE of great help. What you may find, is that you will know the best thing when the time comes, as we often underestimate our subconscious abilities and then of course, there is always the guidance from our unseen friends.

Sealing the Essence

Whenever you create an essence, you can seal it into your Peri- Memory (and intent) at the completion of the harvest process by 'resounding' the vibrations throughout your Peri-Systems. This is done by holding your tongue to the roof of your mouth and contracting the Perineum sharply, three times. Finally, pull the sensation of the vibrations into your lower abdomen and if you wish, say "Thank You", as gratitude is a magical thing!

Testing and Application of Essences

The next activity in the process of creating a usable essence is to commence testing and interpreting the effects of the vibration. Before we look at the actual processes, we shall explore the logic behind the testing process and how, in a Universe where energy acts so diversely, we can be sure that the testing is accurate.

The Effects of an Essence

Our energy (Peri-) systems react with the endless supply of vibrational information we encounter from day to day. Some vibrations have the effect of raising the overall frequency in the Peri- Systems, whilst some lower the overall vibration. So, how does this translate to the actual use of essences in a professional Celtic Reiki environment?

We test each new essence that we harvest in a particular way to discover a 'portrait' of the results it has on us individually and then practise on willing parties to see what the broader effects are. No energy therapy is an exact science; we have such a massive array of frequencies vibrating away in our energy systems, an infinite range of vibrations to choose from when harvesting, and such a personal and unique way of interpreting these that it is more a case of averaging out the effects, rather than being too precise.

As you complete the testing procedure, you will

usually find an assortment of varying, or even conflicting feedback and a few points that correspond – these are the points that you glean for your main prescription notes and the rest is compiled for background reference. With regards to the oral tradition, I offer essence feedback as suggestions when teaching and adhere to that feedback when treating my clients; however I never state that an essence will achieve the same results universally. This leaves other Masters to develop and evolve essences for themselves and maintains the fluidity of the practice. I request that all Celtic Reiki Masters do the same for their students also.

Each vibration we use has particular qualities that work well on specific areas of the client's holistic being. For example, I have found the Essence of 'Green Light' works very well on chest issues, such as asthma, or bronchitis. As Green Light affects the 'heavy vibrations' that are causing dis-ease in this region of the body, it lets the natural vibrations up-shift to a higher level and thus changes the overall frequency of the Peri- Systems and bioenergetic field.

In my own Celtic Reiki practice, this is the case for Green Light, because many of the subjects on whom it was trialled, reported an easing of their chest problems, or chest pain, tightness, etc. on use of the energy. Green Light also influenced many other aspects of a person's being, from emotional calmness to an increased ability to express from the heart, and so on. It is very possible that if a Master were to create a new essence of Green Light and test this for themselves, they may get very different feedback and this is correct for them.

When we test an essence, we are looking for common results in feedback from the particular essence we trigger. These frequent conclusions offer an insight into how and where an essence works and if it is the same for a small group of people, it can be said with confidence that the results will be similar for many others, with some degree of differentiation between individuals. Thus, in my perspective, Green Light helps asthma sufferers in the trial group: it is very likely to help asthma suffers in general. However when used in the field you may find that Green Light will help some sufferers heal entirely, while others have a reduced frequency of attacks and some just desensitise to certain allergens. You may also discover that an individual still has asthma, but becomes very expressive about their emotions! What is important here, is that we have a basis from which to work and can say with some certainty that an essence will work in a set way, although there may be local variations in a treatment environment.

The question often arises of whether an essence can be harmful and thus, what are the consequences of this at the testing and, indeed, harvesting stage. The thing to remember here is that essences are never harmful and if it is not needed, it will have no effect. There may be instances where a person's reaction to an essence seems negative (pain, emotional release, fear, etc.) and special attention should be paid here, as when this occurs it means almost certainly that this is the best essence for the person!

The Methods of Testing

In order to take harvested vibrations that we know very little about and form usable essences that can be specifically prescribed, we require testing, I recommend this is performed in four stages: Intuitive readings, personal testing, general testing, and collation.

By working through this process and producing documentation on what you are using and the results you expect, you are protecting both yourself (legally and morally) and your client, who is getting the best possible care from their Celtic Reiki Master.

The more time you spend on this part of the practice, the better your therapy will be and, hence, the more clients will find their way to you. It is better from standpoint of professional integrity to have 20 solid and documented essences, than 200 that you do not really know what they do! So focus on one essence at a time and gradually introduce more into your practice over time – with the range of existing essences that Masters Calibrate to when training, there is plenty to be going on with!

The First Step: Intuitive Reading

This stage takes two approaches, spontaneous and prompted. The spontaneous approach begins with the harvesting process and includes any thoughts, imagery, or guidance you receive during the harvesting of the essence. This impromptu information can appear at anytime and should always be noted, even if it occurs when the testing has reached completion and you are using the essence in a professional environment.

The prompted information is when you click into Alpha Rhythm and connect with your sub-conscious information about the essence. Considering the fact that our sub-conscious mind is aware of what the energy is doing to our own Peri- Systems, we can confidently state that it can communicate a huge bulk of the information needed to test the essence.

This routine simply includes creating the Alpha Rhythm, asking what the essence does (using any triggers, or a memory of the harvesting) and jotting down any data that is presented back to your conscious mind.

The Second Step: Personal Testing

In conjunction with the intuitive method you can test the essence on yourself as soon as it has been harvested. Indeed, the harvesting process will lead to physical, emotional, mental and spiritual symptoms coming to the surface and these should be noted.

All physical aches, pains, etc. should be recorded about the essence you are working with, along with emotions experienced, thoughts had and any other 'symptom' that comes up. Particular attention can be paid to common themes, as well. For instance, if symptoms tend to be more on the left, or right side of the body, more emotional when listening to music, thinks better in morning, or evening and so on. These will help you to gain an insight into the uses for the essence.

You should be aware when you are working on the essences that the effects can last for several days or longer, so if you want to work on a new essence it is best to wait a few days between using one essence and the next. This will have the effect of dissipating the essence you have been using to a level where it can be 'overwritten' by the new vibrations. This will not 'undo' any benefits of the first, however, as they are working on different layers of the Peri- System.

It is important to take into account at this juncture the difference between the essence you are triggering and the essences of the Peri- System. When a Master triggers a particular essence, this replicates in the Peri- Systems and bioenergetic field of the client. It will affect all information being passed through the various systems, but once the treatment is over, the essence of the client's body will return to normal, with some changes made to specific areas of being. A second essence evoked by the Master will work in the same way, but on different layers, as will a third and so on.

As each new essence affects different layers, the tangible effects caused by changing the frequencies of energy in the Peri- Systems will appear in a day or two and then gradually fade away. In a treatment situation this is all straightforward, however in a testing environment, you should be aware that when you test more than one essence within a three week period, the effects may blur together or blend into each other. So even if you wait a few days, an effect may still be occurring from the previous essence. These similarities can be noted and the symptoms clarified in the general trials stage of the testing process.

The Third Step: General Trials

Once you have tested the essence on yourself it is time to test it on willing subjects who are prepared to experience and feedback any effects from the essence. You should apply only one essence in a three-week period and this will ensure there is no blending of symptoms.

If you applied two essences in the self-testing period that displayed the same symptoms, this is the point to clarify whether the effects were cause by one essence, or both. It is, therefore, a good idea when dealing with two essences that show very similar results to only prescribe one of these to one test subject and find another person to test the second essence. What is important here is to ensure that a case study form is completed for each trial subject and regular feedback is taken throughout the following 21-day period. If your trial participant is willing to keep a journal this is even better!

The Final Step: Collating the Information

When you have gathered all the information from your three trial stages of the testing, you can collate all your information – it is here that the real revelations will really begin to appear as you detect consistencies throughout the information produced. These are the features that you will base your essence applications on and should be recorded for use in a professional environment. You may choose only to list the main similarities in your notes, however all other data should be kept and filed, in case it is needed for future reference.

The Law and Essence Creation

Laws and regulations regarding Reiki practices are different from country to country and are now, also the subject of cultural and religious debate. In most countries Government regulation does not exist, however with some territories now classing Reiki methods as a form of massage, you will need to be aware of the regulations in your particular country.

Now, even if there is no form of regulation, it is, nevertheless, a good idea to record all information from your trials, so that if future laws are passed concerning the self-creation of therapies or essences, you can provide a traceable 'paper-trail' of your processes, findings and professionalism throughout the creation process.

Celtic Reiki Masters are encouraged to work in their individual way and as energetically as possible. This is one area, where you are strongly recommended to keep notes on your Reiki practice, in addition to any other records you have (memory, crystals, etc.). That record can simply be the form of your collated information from trial participants.

Recording Essences

Now that you have completed your trials and compiled all your results, this information can now be recorded in the form of manuals/notes, index cards, crystal, and so on, as discussed previously. These descriptions will be your reference tools in the professional environment and can be used throughout your time as a Master (and teacher) so be sure to start as you mean to go on.

As you start to build up an extensive portfolio of essences, you may find that indexing of symptoms; physical systems, etc. helps in the application process. You will probably find that there are a set number of essences you use over and over again and these will become engrained in your mind. It is however, a good idea to maintain your notes, just in case you need a quick reference guide during a consultation and it is not appropriate to click into Alpha Rhythm.

Combination Essences

If you come across two essences that seem to work on similar, or complementary layers, it is an excellent idea to combine them into one new essence that can be triggered in one go. An example of this could be the essence of 'Minotaur' that works well on helping people through physical and emotional mazes and the essence of Gort, which assists in freeing people from mental/spiritual labyrinths. When combined, the two create an amazing complementary team that work on all layers to help release people when they feel lost, or when being pushed through the maze of life by trauma and upset.

Through this initial connection, we can also distinguish other congruent aspects of this fusion. I have found Minotaur to be mainly 'right hand sided' and Gort to achieve better results on the left hand side of the body, so together they create a balance (this can be seen as a balancing of the right and left hemispheres of the brain). Minotaur releases the past, Gort help perceive a way forward, and so forth.

The process of combining essences is a simple one, which is completed in the Alpha Rhythm, by triggering both energies, one after the other, allowing them both to permeate your Peri- Systems and bioenergetic field, then attaching a new trigger, or giving them a name (in the example above: 'Labyrinth').

You may want to (and it is certainly recommended) carry out new testing processes for the new essence and see how these compare to the individual frequencies. The classifying and recording of your essence will reflect these changes (a plant and concept combination can either remain in 'Concepts', or be placed in the 'Additional' class).

I have discovered that three essences combine to work extremely well together, as trinity, though I'm positive you will find what combinations achieve the best results for you, personally.

Exercises for the Celtic Reiki Master

Traditional Name: HatsuReiHo (Hat-soo-ray-hoe)
Celtic Reiki Name: LlynFawr (Clin-vower)

Task: To cultivate Ki

Technique:

1. Begin by sitting down and relaxing your body
    and mind, close your eyes, ensure that your
    spine is straight and that you are comfortable
    with good back support. Your feet should be
    placed firmly on the floor and your hands
    should be positioned palms down on your lap.
    Now take your attention down to the lower
    abdomen, around 3 to 5 centimetres below your
    belly button, and really explore the sensations
    there while affirming to yourself cerebrally
    that you are about to do LlynFawr.

2. Place your right hand on your left collarbone, with the palm flat against your chest then, in one continuous motion, bring your hand down across your chest and down to the right hip. Do the same motion, but using your left hand on the right shoulder. Complete this stage by repeating the first motion, beginning with right hand on left shoulder.

3. Using the right hand, stroke from the left wrist across the palm and out past the fingers of the left hand. Do this movement again reversing your hands (left hand brushing right hand) and then repeat the original action (right hand brushing left hand).

4. With your hands raised high in the air, palms upwards and fingers pointing directly behind you, connect to the essences of Celtic Reiki. You can do this by visualising the essences as light surging down into your palms, flowing down your arms and into your body, at the same time pull essences up through your feet. As you become aware of the sensations you may feel your arms begin to lower. If you do not feel this, start to lower them anyway. Bring your arms out to the sides 'pulling' the essences around you as if you are creating a bubble around you. Bring the energy/light down past your head and up through your legs, into your body, holding it in your abdomen. Then pull your arms down and around to meet on your lap, palms facing the stomach and your dominant hand closer to the skin.

5. With your hands still on your lap, palms positioned towards your body, focus on the essences that are there. Now place your tongue against the roof of your mouth just behind the top set of teeth and contract the perineum. Breathe in deeply; drawing air into your lower

back and allow your stomach to rise and your chest to expand to the sides. Visualise energy flooding in through your crown and feet, through to your abdomen, gathering there with each in-breath.

6. Now, as you exhale, allow your tongue to fall, relax your perineum and feel the energy flowing out from your abdomen, travelling vigorously from your palms and fingers, your feet and toes. Then repeat the process by inhaling as you did above. You can continue with this technique as long as you like, or is comfortable for you. However, if you begin to feel light headed or faint, stop immediately. This technique should be used with caution by those with high blood pressure or in the latter stages of pregnancy.

7. The next stage is achieved by placing your hands together as if praying and positioned just above the heart centre. A good way of checking if you have the right positioning of the hands is to gently breathe out through the nose, you should be able to feel the breath on your fingertips. Whilst maintaining this position, remember to breathe as in stage 6 unless the contraindications already stated suggest otherwise.

8. Become aware of the place between your middle fingertips. Focus on that space and completely clear your mind of all else. You may find this challenging at first but as each new thought comes into your awareness, just acknowledge it and send it away very calmly then bring your attention back to the place where your middle fingers touch. The more you do this, the more you will learn to just 'be': not only a valuable state for Celtic Reiki practice, but also an incredible state for spiritual enlightenment

Celtic Reiki Name: Craiddseren (Cried-thser-ren)

Task: To increase psychic and intuitive ability

Technique:

1. Sit in a comfortable chair with your feet firmly flat on the floor, your spine straight and your head up. If you wish to play some gentle music, light candles and burn essential oils, this will help create the right ambience required for the exercise.

2. Take a few deep breaths and relax, attempting to release any tension that you are holding. Feel yourself sinking back into the chair yet maintain your straight spine and head up position.

3. Now take your attention to your forehead, lifting your eyes to look at the centre of your forehead, under the closed lids. Keeping this eye position take six slow, deep breaths, each breath lasting six seconds on the inhalation and ten seconds as you exhale. If you cannot do this, take twelve breaths of three seconds for each inhalation and five seconds for each exhalation. With each breath, feel yourself lifting upwards as if you are stretching towards the ceiling of the room.

4. Now place your tongue to the roof of your mouth, just behind the teeth and contract the Perineum. Relax your eyes while continuing to keep them closed. Activate the Celtic Reiki Essences of your choice.

5. Now imagine that you are looking into your head and all is dark except for a small point in the centre of your head. You might want to imagine this point as a star or as a ball of

energy. As you travel towards the light, you want to hone in on the most central point of your head, so that as you get closer, the point becomes smaller and smaller.

6. Maintain this visualisation for several minutes. If at any time during the exercise you feel as if you are falling backwards, go with the sensation and just allow yourself to float 'head over heels' repeatedly.

7. Eventually you reach the central point and bathe in the light. As you just float here in the light, start to immerse yourself in the essences, visualising them all around you, beginning with your hands, feet, head and then travel into the centre of your body. When you are completely immersed in essences, get a real sense of how this feels.

8. Now start to nurture the sense, there is a bubble of Celtic Reiki all around you and this bubble contains all the infinite patterns and dynamics that exist from the perspective of these essences and their source trees, minerals, etc. Start to see these 'unwrapping', as if you are shedding the surface layers away to reveal what is hidden underneath. Start off with one or two individual dynamics (which you could see as threads or lengths of string, maybe even as 'energy onions') and then start to simultaneously unwrap all the dynamics at once, seeing the 'peelings' fall away from you. As you do this, the light gets brighter and brighter; the Reiki more and more powerful.

9. Floating at the centre of your head, unwrapping all the essence dynamics, start to be aware of every single thread/onion/dynamic in existence. Feel each one extending from this central point outwards into the infinite

Universe – never-ending, always flowing. Start to expand outwards along each and every dynamic – reading it, knowing it. Make sure that you expand equally in all directions; taking your time at first to ensure that you are increasing the size of the energy bubble in a uniform way, then becoming faster and faster. Decipher every dynamic equally and at the same time – do not focus on any one dynamic.

10. Continue with this until you recognise the motion/sensation created by travelling along the dynamics and can simply flow with this feeling without thinking about it. Continue this for as long as you wish and then come back into the room.

Celtic Reiki Name: DwrCydio (Dow-r-Kud-dee-oh)

Task: To heighten effect and retention of Celtic Reiki Essences at a Master perspective.

Technique:

1. Start by looking up and to the left, use the trigger, DwrLli (Dow-r-Clee), to activate the essence and then return your eyes to centre.

2. Once you feel the connection to the Celtic Reiki essence, move this sensation to the right side of your head with the assistance of your eyes by looking up and to the right.

3. Trigger a second Celtic Reiki Essence (of your choice), bring it up to the left side of your head and hold it here.

4. Continue to hold the two essences continually and simultaneously for the length of your practice.

5. Upon completion of your practice, switch to DwrTawel (Dow-r-Tah-well) and project this for a further 5 minutes to seal and empower the effects of your practice.

APPENDICES

Appendix A: Finding the right Celtic Reiki Master for your needs & the different modalities of Celtic Reiki

Now that you have seen the various elements and layers of Celtic Reiki practice, let us take a moment to explore the necessary qualities, skills and knowledge a person, looking to train as a Master, should look for. In many ways, this will act as guidelines for all Masters, because what better way of understanding our craft than by recognising what others need from it.

Celtic Reiki has four distinct phases, which vary from Master to Master, although you will be able to conclude what phase a Master teaches from one of these four descriptions:

The Original Celtic Reiki

This is the most commonly found version of Celtic Reiki (or CR as it is often known) and consists of twenty or so essences and basic practices, such as intuitive scanning techniques. These will either be called Reiji Ho, Byosen, etc. or renamed with Celtic/Welsh/Gaelic titles. There are usually three attunements and these are usually conducted remotely. Aided by the Internet, this version of Celtic Reiki spread across the globe very quickly and is often slotted into 'attunement websites' – sites that offer energy therapies with the emphasis on attunement, as opposed to professional practice. Prices range from free of charge, up to and around $75 and can be found easily by searching the web for 'Celtic Reiki' or even on eBay!

Adapted Celtic Reiki

This later version of Celtic Reiki is based on the Original version, yet it has been adapted either by myself or other Celtic Reiki Masters. These adaptations can be as simple as additional essences and renaming of techniques, to vast transformations of the practice with greater emphasis on diverse fields of practice or philosophy. I have encountered versions of Celtic Reiki with a greater grounding in Celtic mythology, Druidic elements, Wiccan practices, and other cultural influences, such as Native American and Mayan wisdom. These can be found via an Internet search and the individual Masters will be able to explain what emphases their modality has. Prices, once again, range from around $25 to $150+ and vary in attunements and course materials, etc.

I would advise you to choose the Celtic Reiki modality that you are most resonant with – if you practise Wicca, for example, an adaptation with Wiccan influences would be good for you, and so on. I actively encourage adaptation, flexibility and individuality in Celtic Reiki practice, however, do be aware that some Masters refer to their adaptations with an approach that suggests their methodology is more powerful or in some way 'better' than anybody else's. I have also seen marketing that hints the adaptation process is 'exclusive' to a particular modality. All Masters adapt their practice, either in major ways or with little nuances – the issue here is that no modality is better than any other – it boils down to resonance with the individual Apprentice.

Celtic Reiki 2005

In 2005, I completely re-imagined my Celtic Reiki system to strip away the Usui Reiki principles and create a system based on the Shinto perspective of Reiki. This also included an increase in Celtic spirituality, the introduction of the oral tradition in practice and teaching, and many other enhancements to the system. This iteration of Celtic Reiki and the adaptations based upon it are less likely to be found on the Internet, as they are favoured by professional therapists and teachers who work on a face-to-face basis. With one or two-day workshops, people are guided through Celtic Reiki with an emphasis on treatment and mentoring in a regulated way. These Masters tend to have accreditation from the nrg organisation and adhere to the fluidity principle of adaptation as a personal preference.

Prices for these classes are usually from $150 upwards and your Master will be able to provide you with information about their qualification, lineage, insurance and accreditation, etc. I would recommend this form of training to anybody who wants to be sure of being eligible for professional insurance and to work in line with the increasing regulation in the 'Energy Therapy Industry'.

Celtic Reiki 2009

The 2009 version of Celtic Reiki was vast in subject matter, range of practice and sheer immersion for those using it. With hundreds of essences, shaping and styling practices, various treatment methods and psychic ability training, Avatars, Realms, Lores, a broadening of cultural philosophies and deeper understanding of oral traditions, Lost Language, and many other factors, Celtic Reiki became richer in scope and experience.

I feel the need to reiterate here, these adaptations are not better—they are different. Since 2009 Celtic Reiki is intentionally more complex than earlier methods, because I wanted to create a greater sense of commitment to their abilities for Masters.

With increasing regulation and decreasing standards of teaching, I wanted to readdress the challenges we face in the world of energy work from a professional point of view and I wanted to share an experience with others. As opposed to isolated chunks of teaching, practice, energy, attunement, etc,. I wanted a fully integrated adventure for people to enjoy, experience and lose themselves in.

Most of all, I wanted to create a realm where Masters felt confident to unleash their potential, to trust their instincts and abilities, to adapt with integrity to offer the ultimate care for their students and clients.

Celtic Reiki 2013

In 2013, Celtic Reiki experienced a further core-shift. The increasing polarity between the behaviour of certain Reiki Therapists across the globe, changes in legislation and regulation in different territories, and the needs both of better professionalism within our community and more profound results for our clients, meant that a radical approach was necessary.

At this juncture, I made the decision to only accredit licensed Realm Masters for teaching, who were prepared to uphold the quality of service and latest iterations of our therapy. With so many changes and adaptations over the years I could only, in good conscience, offer my approval to those who I knew were acting with integrity and in-depth knowledge. This was achieved through assessment and certification that all Realm Masters must take to qualify for teaching others.

Yet, further changes were taking place within Celtic Reiki as it became an art that expended way beyond healing. Detailed profiling tools opened the way for new treatment methods; those which focus upon emotional trauma, childhood experiences, superstition and control memes, legacy, skills and perspective, and many other areas of influence.

The introduction of two extensive Realm Master book also increased the the level of knowledge and wisdom imparted to Realm Masters beyond this point. These two immense tomes present an insight into each Realm and Mystic, as well as revealing the secrets behind Celtic Reiki and various new Mystics and Realms of discovery. These include The Seer and The Lost Realms.

Celtic Reiki 2016 and Beyond

With the advent of One Therapy, Celtic Reiki continues to evolve into a greater methodology. The Earth element in a series of therapeutic relationships; Celtic Reiki now exists as part of a greater system—one that includes vReiki, The Viridian Method, Karmic Regression Therapy, and vPsychic.

One Therapy integrates space, time, perspective, experience, and dimension. Augmenting our Celtic Reiki with other therapies gives Realm Masters a vast array of new skills.

You can find out more about Celtic Reiki Masters who train others to the latest version of Celtic Reiki on the mPowr website at www.celtic-reiki.com

There are also forms of energy practice titled 'Celtic Wisdom Reiki', 'Celtic Energies Therapy', 'Celtic Energies Reiki' and so on. These are not Celtic Reiki based and whilst have validity in their own right, they should not be confused with Celtic Reiki practice.

If you are unsure as to the validity of a Celtic Reiki Master, ask to see their Realm Master certification, their license number, and for their lineage, which should begin with me (Martyn Pentecost) as the Originator and work on from there.

Appendix B: Sample Essence Harvest Form

Harvest of essence (Name):

Date/Time Harvest Completed:

Reference:
(Choose a reference to connect with any future harvesting of the same subject)

Essence Used:
(Name of Archetypal Essence used in Harvest)

Label:
(The label you attached during harvest to re-trigger essence)

Feedback from Harvest:
(Sensory information, or intuitive response to harvest)

Appendix C: Sample Testing Case Study Form
Subject Name:

Address:

Contact Telephone Number:

Name of Doctor:
Contact details of Doctor:

Date of essence application:

Any reoccurring health issues:
Prescribed Medication:
Additional Information:
Name of Essence Applied:
Master's Feedback from Treatment:
Subject's Feedback from Treatment:
Follow-up information (Date & Feedback):

Bibliography

Energy Medicine, James Oschman
(Churchill Livingstone, 978-0443062612)

Molecules of Emotion, Candace B. Pert
(Simon & Schuster, 978-0684846347)

Brain Sense, Faith Hickman Brynie
(Amacom, 978-0814413241)

The Spirit of Reiki, Walter Lubeck, et al
(Lotus Press, 978-0914955672)

Supernature:
A Natural History of the Supernatural, Lyall Watson
(Coronet, 978-0340188330)

The Silva Mind Control Method, Jose Silva
(Mass Market, 978-0671739898)

The Celtic Reiki Home Experience

If you would like to experience the wonder of Celtic Reiki Mastership with Martyn Pentecost, you can discover the rich and immersive adventure of the mPowr Celtic Reiki Home Experience at http://www.celtic-reiki.com.

Also by Martyn Pentecost & published by mPowr:

The Official Guide to Celtic Reiki:
A Walk in the Forest
ISBN: 978-1907282003

Celtic Reiki: Stories from the Sacred Grove
ISBN: 978-1907282010

Karmic Regression Therapy & Karmic Reiki:
An Official Guide
ISBN: 978-1907282034

vPsychic
ISBN: 978-1907282041

vPsychic Adventures
ISBN: 978-1907282058

The Little Book of Celtic Reiki Wisdom
ISBN: 978-1907282317

Bedtime Stories from the Woodland
ISBN: 978-1907282232

The Key
ISBN: 978-1907282171

The Key in Your Pocket
ISBN: 978-1907282447

Legacy
ISBN: 978-1907282485

CPSIA information can be obtained
at www.ICGtesting.com
Printed in the USA
FSOW01n1145181116
27558FS

9 781907 282027